WHAT PEOPLE ARE SA

SEASONAL AWAR
WELLBEI

This book is a gem! If you're looking for a truly novel approach to changing and improving your life, look no further.

Jonny Bowden, PhD, CNS

The Rogue Nutritionist and author of *The 150 Healthiest Foods on Earth*

An innovative and well-documented approach is needed for anyone who wishes to improve wellbeing using natural methods; such a strategy respecting seasons is hugely clever and promising.

Dr Georges Mouton, Internationally-renowned pioneer of Functional Medicine, author of *Dr Mouton's Methods* and *The Intestinal Ecosystem and Optimal Health*

I love the seasonal format, which makes this book so easy to read and digest. It is invaluable to teachers, health and beauty practitioners, and nutritionists - as well as those wishing to lose weight. Well researched and written, this should be on everyone's bookshelf.

Dawn Cragg, MBE, CIDESCO, BABTAC, International authority on beauty

Seasonal Awareness and Wellbeing

Looking and Feeling Better the Easy Way

Seasonal Awareness and Wellbeing

Looking and Feeling Better the Easy Way

Marie-Claire Wilson

Winchester, UK
Washington, USA

First published by O-Books, 2011
O-Books is an imprint of John Hunt Publishing Ltd., Laurel House, Station Approach,
Alresford, Hants, SO24 9JH, UK
office1@o-books.net
www.o-books.com

For distributor details and how to order please visit the 'Ordering' section on our website.

ISBN: 978 1 84694 469 7

A CIP catalogue record for this book is available from the British Library.

Design: Stuart Davies

Printed in the UK by CPI Antony Rowe
Printed in the USA by Offset Paperback Mfrs, Inc

CONTENTS

To my partner Stan

Acknowledgments

I would like to thank everyone who has supported me whilst writing, directly and indirectly. Special thanks to:

My aunt, Gracia, for lending me her lovely seasons diary, which was a source of inspiration

My friend, Sarah for providing helpful comments on the Introduction, despite working 12 hour shifts and living on a different continent

Gill Haines, who has provided brilliant advice and mentoring on many of my wellbeing projects

Chris Lyon, who taught me art in secondary school, for creating the beautiful illustrations

My friend and colleague Dina for her amazing remedial massages that undid the damage caused by hours in front of the computer

My dad, John, for his encouragement

My mum Maria-Rosa and step-dad Terry for their enthusiasm in the project and for providing a quiet place to write with a well-stocked fridge - also to the kittens for not causing too much trouble, and my mum (again) for organising the illustrations

My partner, Stan for reading the whole text and providing many useful comments and for his ongoing support, patience and understanding, without which the book would not have been completed

Introduction

The inspiration for this book came from my observations of how the seasons affect wellbeing. I believe that some of the more negative impacts of the seasons can be prevented through awareness of the shifts in nature, and that certain lifestyle changes have greater effects when made at particular times of year. For example, in the UK, January is generally considered a dull and miserable month, due to post-festive hangovers, broken New Year's resolutions and poor weather. Through rethinking ideas about winter and making small, rather than drastic steps towards improving diet and lifestyle, it is possible to have an entirely different experience in January. Early spring, on the other hand, is a good time to make lifestyle changes, as it is a period of growth and change, and adopting new habits in March or April, means they are a part of life and are producing results by the time the distractions of the summer arrive.

In researching this book, I have enjoyed discovering more about seasonal traditions, parts of which still exist today. I wanted to blend concepts of these traditions and changes in nature, with practical, yet holistic, approaches to wellbeing, fitness and weight loss.

The chapters represent the development of a theme, but it is not necessary to start at January and work through the year - some topics are re-visited throughout the book in slightly different ways. I begin in January, thinking of the reader as someone ready to start on a new path; each month progress is made and their lifestyle plan is considered from a slightly different angle. My book is also intended as a tool for people who already pay attention to their lifestyle, and who merely want to make some positive changes or explore a fresh approach. Some topics, such as contraception and sleep, can be taken out of the seasonal context, and the "Workbook" sections at the end of each chapter are aimed at encouraging readers to record their thoughts and create their own plan.

I have focused on the climate and cultural practices of England, which is where I live, with references to other parts of the British Isles. The content is however, directly relevant to any country with a colder, darker winter, a warmer, brighter summer and intermediate periods - in the Southern Hemisphere, the autumn and winter concepts would be useful from April to August, for example. Some practices from other cultures are included, but these are not in-depth studies, and are added to provide comparison and flavour.

As Christianity has been the official religion of England for over a thousand years, many of the customs referred to are linked to this religion. The book does not have a Christian theme though, and could be helpful to people from all faiths.

If you are looking for a way to feel and look better, that works in harmony with nature and the body, I hope you will find this book useful and enjoyable. If you would like to connect with me and with other readers, please see the Seasonal Awareness and Wellbeing Book Facebook page, or you can contact me directly.

Best wishes,
Marie-Claire.

www.bodyprogresscentre.com
mc@bodyprogresscentre.com
@BPC_Wellbeing

A note about supplements

I have mentioned the scientific basis for selecting nutritional supplements throughout the book. Most studies are imperfect, and the results of molecular analysis may have relatively little bearing on an individual's daily life. Also, it would be possible to find studies that perhaps refute the established arguments for and against a particular supplement being effective. However, I prefer to work with some kind of reference point when choosing and recommending supplements.

If a particular study concludes that a supplement is no more effective than a placebo, or if no research has been carried out on a supplement, this does not mean it is immediately useless for everyone. There are many reasons why trials may not be carried out on such products in the first place, and then why data might be interpreted in a certain manner. Additionally, individuals vary in their biochemical responses. Equally, a supplement that is well supported by research will not necessarily be effective for everyone who tries it. My view is that a supplement that has been the subject of a number of trials, and which has returned positive results, is simply more likely to work for a given individual. An un-researched supplement or a product that has given negative results in a specified group of people is less likely to be effective.

Whilst I hope this book will help its readers to feel better and achieve their goals in terms of weight loss and fitness, it is not intended to treat any disease, and is not a substitute for a consultation with a doctor or other health-care or wellbeing professional. Please consult with your doctor before making lifestyle changes, including starting supplements. Be aware that some supplements and herbs can interact with each other, and with prescription medication.

January

New Year, New You?

For centuries, 1 January has been associated with making a new start – after the winter solstice, the days slowly begin to lengthen, and this has always been a cause for celebration. The English "January" is named after Janus, the two-headed Roman god of gates, who looks simultaneously to the past and to the future, so reviewing the year's progress and making changes during this month – such as eating more healthily or exercising regularly – would seem fitting

Despite the promise of renewal linked with the New Year, and the change in the direction of the sun (or rather the change in the tilt of the Earth on its axis), January is deepest winter, a time when much of nature is suspended. The Christian celebration of the birth of Jesus at midwinter may have echoes in older religions focusing on the sun. The symbolism of the birth of a powerful being in the form of a helpless infant is significant – like the sun at this time of year, the child must gain in strength before it can cause direct change. This is an opportunity to balance the concept of new starts with the facts of winter.

After the Christmas and New Year holidays, the start of January was traditionally connected with preparation. In England, it saw the start of ploughing – in some areas marked by a festival, with plough games, religious services and the collection of money.

This January then, rather than opting for a dramatic new start, take the opportunity to prepare. Whilst health and fitness resolutions are something of a nationally-recognised custom, unfortunately, so is giving up on them after a few weeks. By harmonising with the more static energy of the season, it is possible to increase the chances of making progress in the longer term, without feeling that healthy living is difficult.

Checklist – understanding how the time of year affects you

Consider the following – if you answer "yes" to more than one question, it is unlikely that you will benefit from attempting large diet and lifestyle changes in January/winter.

- Do you tend to feel more tired in winter?
- Does your mood tend to be lower in winter – no matter what else is happening in your life? (See February chapter for tips on supplements to support mood)
- Would you say you suffer from SAD or winter blues?
- Do you have more intense carbohydrate cravings in winter?
- Does the post-Christmas period often involve financial restriction? Do you try to make savings on food?
- Does colder weather lead you to eat more rich foods?
- Do you find winter difficult or unpleasant?

The problem with January resolutions

It is of course possible stick to New Year's resolutions and achieve the desired results – a slimmer physique, better energy levels, improved habits. Often, though, this "success against the odds" can reinforce negative ideas about about healthy eating, losing weight (fat) and exercise. After the excesses of the festive season, typically "healthy" food seems boring, and exercise in winter is often a chore. Losing weight at a time of year when energy should be conserved is generally unpleasant.

If healthy behaviours do not feel natural, it is unlikely that they will be continued consistently in the longer term. Using January to commit to making positive changes, and to start preparing for action, rather than new habits, will help to set a more sustainable pattern; ceasing to see January frugality as the flip-side of festive excess will help to challenge "all or nothing" behaviour (see December chapter).

For non-beginners

For those who already have an exercise or nutrition plan, or who are not focused on losing weight (fat), January is not the right month to increase intensity or focus on breaking a plateau in the gym. Use the period of relative stasis to re-consider your goals, using the space at the end of this chapter as a guide and saving action for a little later.

Do not try to reverse any "damage" done by festive season overindulgence this January, but consider how exercise and healthy food choices can remain a key part of life for the remainder of the winter.

Exercise

- List what can be done to ensure continuation of exercise, without it becoming a chore – examples include taking gym kit to work and having lunchtime workouts, including weekend exercise sessions or including some well-designed, challenging home-based training routines
- Experiment with new ideas to prevent boredom – try a class, learn to skip, or add in some interval training. Focus on the variety and stimulation, rather than making large changes
- For those that exercise seriously, January might be a good time to review goals and progress with a Personal Trainer or Strength Coach. Focus on technique to begin with, leaving the push on performance until later in the year

Nutrition

- The list of Realistic New Year's Resolutions on the following pages may help with identification of areas where unhelpful foods and drinks may creep in to an otherwise healthy diet. Eliminate excess alcohol, and increase awareness of social situations involving unhealthy snacks

- Focus on maintaining a varied diet, rather than cutting foods out – make an effort to eat a variety of different coloured vegetables every day, and to drink plenty of good quality water

Rethinking your approach to food

During the festive season, eating to be sociable, to fit with tradition and to relieve boredom and frustration is common. In January, examine your general approach to food, and to begin to align it with your goals. This does not need to involve large changes to routines – simply increasing awareness of which foods are eaten, how and when is sufficient for now.

Use the following questions to highlight aspects of your approach to food.

1. I stop eating when I am full
a) Always
b) Mostly
c) Sometimes
d) Not really – I often overeat and then feel uncomfortable

2. I take pleasure in my food
a) Always
b) When I have time
c) Not really – I see food mainly as a fuel source

3. When eating I give my full attention to the meal
a) Always
b) Sometimes
c) Never – I don't have time for that

4. I eat at my desk/workspace
a) Never
b) Only in exceptional circumstances

c) Occasionally
d) Frequently

What your answers mean: These four questions relate to your the attention you give to your meals. Realising when to stop eating sounds simple, but many people continue to eat after being physically full. This is more likely when eating in a hurry or whilst being engaged in another activity, when meals are only once or twice a day, or when eating for emotional reasons. Sometimes it is only after a pause in eating that fullness is felt. Also, there are the cultural aspects – it is often considered rude or wasteful to leave food on the plate. For those that find it hard to stop until all the food has disappeared, use a smaller plate and take smaller servings. Slow down and minimise distractions – this will help you to recognise the feeling of fullness. It is also worth making time – even 10 minutes - to focus on eating, rather than eating whilst working or surfing the internet.

5. There are certain foods/drinks I would find it difficult to live without
a) Yes – I need my coffee/wine/chocolate/bread to get through the day!
b) No – I prefer some foods over others, but don't feel I am dependent on particular foods

What your answer means: Most of us prefer some foods over others, but feeling unable to do without a certain food can lead to unhealthy habits and can be the sign of an imbalance. Breaking an "addiction" may require avoiding the food completely for a short period. A few weeks without sweet foods, for example, means that cravings may actually decrease, even when sweets are re-introduced.

6. Throughout the day my energy levels are:

a) Generally stable
b) Mildly fluctuating – there is a tendency towards the mid-afternoon dip, but generally it is manageable
c) Dramatically fluctuating – I rely on caffeine and sugar to help me through dips

What your answer means: Fluctuating levels of energy can signify blood sugar imbalances. Refined and simple carbohydrates such as desserts, white bread and commercial cereals are processed quickly by the body, causing a rapid rise in the amount of sugar in the blood. The body reacts to this by releasing insulin, the storage hormone, which causes entry of sugar in the blood to cells, where it can be used as fuel, or stored as fat. So initially, after eating refined or simple carbohydrates, you might have an energy boost, but as sugar is removed from the blood and stored in cells, a "crash" can be experienced, with tiredness and edginess. Eating fewer refined carbohydrates can help to keep blood sugar levels more consistent, meaning more stable energy levels throughout the day.

7. Which of the following is most like you?
a) I think in advance about meals and snacks, prepare as much as possible and generally make the best choices I can (although this does not work out 100% of the time)
b) Planning what I eat is not an option for me – mostly I grab whatever I can, when I have the time
c) How I eat depends a lot on my mood. Sometimes I can plan meals and eat healthily, at other times I eat for comfort, or out of boredom
d) How I eat depends on my situation – when I can control my food, I do, but I often end up eating unhealthily when I am with others, or away on holiday, for example
e) Food is one of my main sources of enjoyment – I like to spend time cooking and eating

f) I eat in a certain way, and can't see this changing unless absolutely necessary
g) Controlling what and how I eat is important to me, and I make sure that nothing gets in the way of my plans

What your answer means: Most people eat for reasons other than physical sustenance. Understanding your patterns can help to identify any unhealthy behaviours, and with motivation it is possible to address these. For example, eating out of boredom or for comfort can be tackled by using other methods to enhance mood. It is also unhealthy to have an approach to eating that is too controlled – thinking of food only as a combination of nutrients is stressful, and means missing out on the joy of good meals.

Realistic New Year's Resolutions to start from 1 January
The focus now should be on small lifestyle changes that feel easy to make – but which may have a noticeable and lasting impact. The following practical and simple ideas relating to food will help anyone looking to feel better or lose weight.

Cut down on alcohol
After the festive season, many people choose to cut down on alcohol, and this is a "typical" resolution that should be considered, perhaps also for the longer term. Think about restricting alcohol to weekends, or even to special occasions such as birthdays and Valentine's day.

Advantages:
- Alcohol has many negative effects on the body, one of which being that whilst alcohol is present, fat cannot be used as fuel, as the body prioritises removal of the alcohol
- People tend to make poor food choices under the influence of alcohol and hangovers the following day can lead to

reduced physical activity and further poor food choices
- Cutting down on alcohol will also save money, which could be invested in good quality food. It may also help to improve the quality of your sleep

What might be difficult about doing this:
- Social pressures – many social gatherings in our culture are centred on alcohol, and staying sober whilst others are drunk means being left out
- If you enjoy alcoholic drinks for their own sake - there is no need to give up, simply restrict quantity and/or frequency

Break the latte/cappuccino and muffin habit
A common reason behind unwanted weight gain and its longer term health consequences is that treats, which should be occasional occurrences, become daily habits. Having a pastry at a coffee shop once in a while is unlikely to impact a person's health or shape, but the habit of a cappuccino and a muffin every day could make it difficult to lose weight (fat). This does not mean giving up either coffee or desserts. Switching to americano coffee (ideally black, or with a splash of milk) or tea, and saving up real treats for the end of the week, for example, will make a difference.

Advantages:
As long as the lack of coffee shop treats is not compensated for with other unhealthy snacks, simply cutting down pastries, desserts and sweet beverages consumed out of habit could contribute significantly towards weight (fat) loss, as well as saving money

What might be difficult about doing this:
- Peer pressure – coffee and cake might be part of the

culture at a particular work place. Simply changing the choice of drinks and snacks may help, as may suggesting a new work ritual, such as visiting a specialist tea shop

Take meals and snacks to work

Chocolate, crisps and sandwiches are always readily available, and many people turn to these whilst at work or on the go. Solve this problem with a little planning, bring leftover dinner to work, and keep snacks available during the day.

Advantages:

- Cutting out sweet snacks and ready-prepared food is key to achieving and maintaining a healthy weight
- This is another area where a healthier approach is more cost effective

What might be difficult about doing this:

- Position at work - this might mean it is unacceptable to bring in tubs of food from home. Bring your own snacks, and investigate local restaurants/cafes for healthy lunch options
- Lack of fridge or food heating facilities – if a case can't be made for changing this, stick to non-perishables

Make healthier choices for comfort foods

Foregoing warming, comforting foods in winter is not necesssary – typical comfort foods can be replaced by healthier options.

Ideas for comfort food swaps:

- Swap crisps and fried chips with home-made root vegetable "crisps"
- Swap tinned baked beans with home-cooked bean dishes (e.g., Mexican style black beans), or other forms of tinned beans without added sugar, such as refried pinto beans

- Swap chocolate ice cream for Booja-Booja "Stuff in a Tub" – less impact on blood sugar (but high in fructose, so this is not something that should be part of your diet every day)
- Swap highly sweetened chocolate bars with many additives for good quality, organic, dark chocolate or raw chocolate products
- Swap pasta and white rice as meal bases for brown rice and quinoa

Advantages:

- Enjoying the experience of warming, tasty food without worrying about the effect on healthy eating programmes

What might be difficult about doing this:

- Resisting the temptation to eat twice as much

The language of weight loss

Calories

Calories are an integral part of the language of weight loss and healthy eating, and many people do achieve their weight loss goals through counting calories, at least in the short term. However, there may be too much focus placed on calories as a method of evaluating food.

A calorie is a unit of energy equal to the amount of heat required to raise the temperature of one kilogram of water by one degree at one atmosphere pressure, and explained this way it seems to have relatively little bearing on physiology. The caloric content of a food is determined by burning it in a bomb calorimeter and observing temperature change, which is not how the human body works. This means that the calorie content of a food determined in this way may have minimal relation to the effect on the body, as food has diverse effects on hormones and neurotransmitters, and is not simply used as fuel for an engine.

Depending on the type of food, the same quantity of calories could have a very different effect on mood, energy levels and tendency to store fat – 100 calories' worth of lean meat will not have the same metabolic effects as a 100 calorie "diet" chocolate bar. The meat has a greater satiating effect, and less of an impact on insulin, the storage hormone, which affects fat gain. It also contains useful vitamins and minerals. The chocolate has few nutritional benefits, unless it is a high quality dark chocolate bar that retains the antioxidant effects of cocoa, and strongly stimulates insulin because of its sugar content, meaning excess glucose not used up immediately is stored, potentially as fat.

Whilst eating 10,000 calories per day, no matter the source, would lead to fat gain for most people, assessment of food should not be based on calorie content alone. Additionally, calorie control, portion control and food weighing all lead to the same conclusion – that food is inherently wrong and that its intake should be minimised. This is not the case, and by choosing the right foods it is possible to feel and look better, whilst still enjoying tasty meals.

Glycaemic Index (GI) and Insulin Index (II)

The glycaemic index of a food refers to how quickly it causes an increase in the sugar level of the blood. Refined and simple carbohydrates, which are rapidly converted into glucose (the main sugar used by the body), have high GIs, as they quickly and dramatically impact the blood sugar level. Proteins and fats have much lower GIs, as they cause little increase in blood sugar. Consumption of high GI foods can lead to fluctuating energy levels, as well as to fat gain, because changes to the blood sugar level stimulates the release of insulin, the storage hormone. Insulin allows sugar in the blood to be used as fuel by cells, but once immediate energy requirements have been met, it causes the excess sugar to be stored as glycogen in the muscles (the storage form of glucose) or as fat.

Most foods which cause rapid rises in GI, cause proportionate changes in the amount of insulin released (high II as well as high GI), as would be expected. There are some foods, such as dairy products, which have low GI ratings, but high insulin indices.

GI and II are more useful concepts when choosing foods than calories, although too much focus should not be placed on the GI scores of individual foods either. White potatoes, for example, have a relatively high GI, and are therefore excluded from many fat loss plans. Eaten alone, they are a high GI meal, but this is not the case when they are combined in small quantities with lower GI foods such as meat, fibrous vegetables and healthy fats.

Weight loss and fat loss

The term "weight loss" is used widely, and is used in this book, but it is important to keep in mind that weight loss goals are in fact fat loss goals. The two do overlap – losing fat means losing weight, but it is also possible to lose significant amounts of fat without much impact on the reading on the scales, if a person is also exercising and building muscle, and conversely, it is possible to lose weight, but not fat.

Building muscle can cause an increase in weight, but this is very different from the weight gain associated with increased levels of fat. Body Mass Index (BMI), which gives a measure of how heavy a person is for their height, is a useful concept, but can be misleading. Two equally tall women weighing 65kg (so having the same BMI) could be in very different situations in terms of health and appearance, depending on the ratio of muscle to fat – one may look slim and sporty and be healthy and strong, whilst the other may be unfit and carrying an unhealthy amount of weight as fat. Therefore, do not rely on weight to provide information on progress, and do not feel discouraged if despite exercising and eating well, the scales do not change - you may well be losing fat but building muscle. Focus more on how you feel, inch loss, clothing size and body fat percentage. (If having your body fat percentage assessed, use calliper methods as impedance machines are far less accurate).

It is also worth considering that very rapid weight loss is not usually fat loss. Weight is more easily lost as water, or from glycogen stores, or even muscle, than as fat. Whilst in the initial phases of a fat loss plan, changes can occur quite quickly, continued true fat loss requires long-term commitment.

Starting an exercise plan

Most people lead sedentary lives, and planning in exercise is important for health. For increasing levels of movement in January, focus on enjoyable activities – most likely, these will be indoors. January is not the best month to begin a new exercise programme or increase the intensity of an existing one, but if you wish to join a gym, see the Resources section for a guide on making your choice. Check with your doctor that it is safe to increase your activity levels, and consider the following gym-free ideas:

- Design a body weight programme for yourself including skipping, lunges, squats and press ups. These can all be performed at home. Better still - engage a good Personal Trainer to design and review the programme and your progress
- Start attending an enjoyable but relatively intense exercise class, such as Body Pump or Boxercise
- Take up a team sport, considering whether it can be played indoors as well as outdoors
- Try out exercise DVDs, adding a few simple pieces of equipment such as resistance bands or dumbells to increase intensity

- Winter is an important time for conservation activities, so consider getting involved in local projects. Working with other people will take the focus away from the cold, and you will also have the sense of achievement that comes from having made a difference to your local environment
- Make activity part of your day. Taking the stairs instead of the lift and getting off the bus a stop earlier will not change your body shape, but could help boost metabolism and energy levels if done regularly

Running

Men and women braving the cold for an early morning/evening run is a common sight in January. Running is a versatile, low cost form of exercise that can be performed alone or as part of a running club, and which also allows connection with nature.

Despite its popularity, running may not be the best option for weight (fat) loss. Long duration low intensity exercise (i.e., that continues for more than 45 minutes) can lead to increases in cortisol, the stress hormone – which encourages fat storage. Also, whilst it may be true that at lower intensities, most calories used come from fat, the body will also use muscle, rather than fat, as a fuel once carbohydrate stores have been exhausted, and the total number of calories used is in any case small. More importantly, once the exercise session has finished, the metabolic rate does not remain increased. This is in contrast to resistance training, which is actually more effective for weight (fat) loss due to the post-workout increases in the metabolic rate, required to repair the muscles.

If improved fitness is your goal, again, running may not be the best option – exercising at a steady pace does not challenge the body sufficiently, and after a few weeks of making gains, a plateau may be reached. It is also important to pay close attention to the choice of footwear and to technique when running, as these can be sources of injuries.

Overall, those keen to run should keep sessions short, and should try to include interval sprints within sessions, where possible. A progressive programme should be designed, and some resistance-type work should be included, even if this is a home-based workout.

What else to consider in January

Consider wider health and wellbeing goals this January. Some ideas:

- Request specialised equipment at work to help prevent musculoskeletal problems. This may include trackball mice, back supports, foot rests and equipment to raise a laptop to eye height
- Take steps to create a more sleep-friendly bedroom. De-clutter, add darker curtains or try out an eye mask (see April chapter for more information on sleep)
- Have a deep tissue massage or acupuncture to help with musculoskeletal aches and pains. Research practitioners first, or go by recommendations, as the quality of treatment can vary widely. Some clinics allow clients to pay what they can afford, and it is possible to be medically referred for some treatments, or to have them covered by health insurance
- Book a GP appointment to discuss health concerns such as low energy – this could be due to thyroid problems or anaemia, for example (see February chapter)
- Book a family planning appointment to review contraceptive choices (see May chapter)
- Get in touch with old friends – social contact can influence hormones and neurotransmitters
- Make a PMS action plan, starting with the information in this book (see May chapter)
- Decrease the allergic potential of your home – remove or

reduce carpets and soft furnishings
- Book a dentist or hygienist appointment
- Book an eye test – headaches whilst using a computer may be due to long-sightedness

Chapter summary

- View January as a time of preparation, and make simple, rather than drastic changes - the body requires nurturing and rest during winter
- Start to examine your approach to food and work on easily-identifiable unhelpful habits, such as overindulgence in alcohol, or treats that have become daily occurrences
- Start increasing activity levels – focus on enjoyable activities (no need to join a gym)

Workbook section

General plan for the year

My health and wellbeing/fitness/weight loss goals for this year are:

Why this is important to me:

What has stopped me achieving my goals in the past:

What I am going to change about my life to achieve my goals this year:

Food

Exercise

Attitudes
Habits/routines

Other health and wellbeing issues I would like to change this year, with ideas for addressing them:

January
How I usually feel in January:

Steps I will take regarding what and how I eat in January:

Steps I will take to increase activity in January:

Other plans for January:

Spring

Reawakening
Change
New Starts

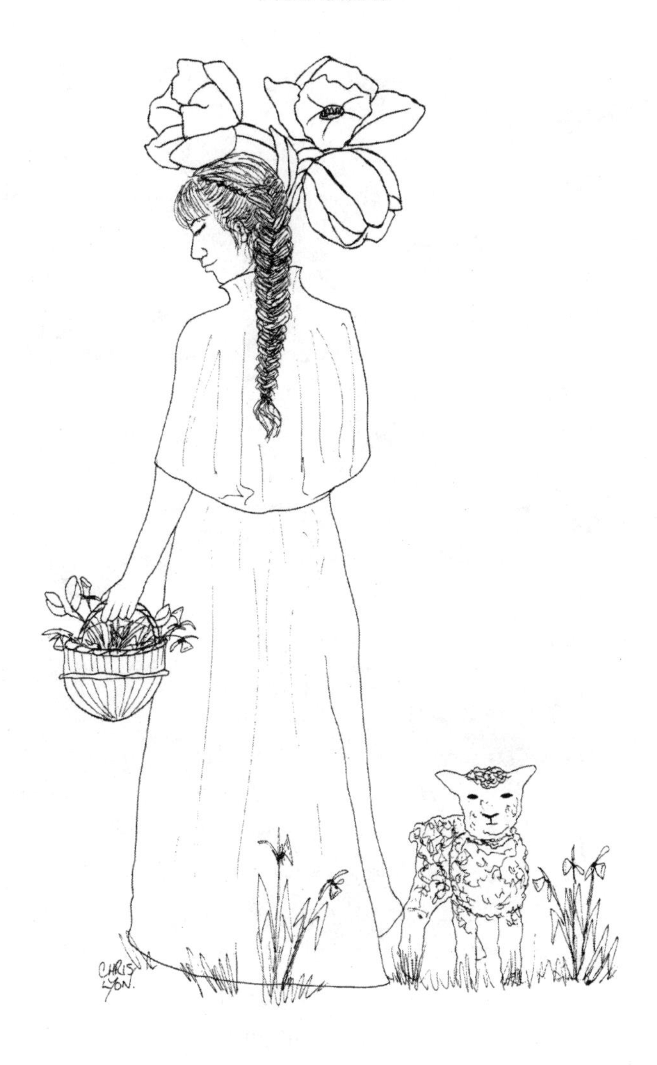

February

Entertain yourself!

By February, winter seems endless, with continuing grey, cold weather and long nights. In the past though, this time was considered the start of spring. Farming communities would have started moving livestock from winter pastures to make way for sowing, and according to the Venerable Bede, the Anglo-Saxons offered cakes to their deities during the month equivalent to February, perhaps in the hope of the fields being fertile and able to yield a good harvest.

The pre-Christian Gaelic feast of Imbolc on 1 February, corresponding to the lactation of ewes, marked the opening of the new season in Ireland. The date of the festival later became associated with the most important Irish female saint, St Brigid, who may have been a Christian representation of an earlier pagan goddess. St Brigid's night activities involved a family meal, and the making of offerings, in the form of food, drink or woven crosses or dolls. The cult of Brigid was visible only in Ireland and areas of Irish influence.

In Britain, Candlemas was the feast that took place in early February (2 February). It is a feast of purification and light, believed to be linked to the presentation of the infant Jesus as the "light of the world" at the temple, and the purification rites his mother Mary would have needed to undergo 6 weeks after giving birth. Interestingly, February was also seen as a time of purification in ancient Rome, with the name of the month coming from the Februa or Februatio ritual,which celebrated the cleansing properties of water and the expedition of the end of winter.

A key part of the original Candlemas celebrations in Britain was the blessing and lighting of candles, and after the Reformation, the feast was pared down as blessing candles was seen to belong to the superstitions of Roman Catholicism. For a while, an opportunity to celebrate in early February was provided by the feast days of saints such as St Crispin and St Blaise, but now St Valentine's Day is the only widely acknowledged feast during the month.

Whilst there were a number of Christian martyrs named Valentine, one of whom is thought to have died on 14 February, there is no evidence connecting any of the original St Valentines with concepts of romantic love. However, Valentine's day has been an opportunity for love and wooing for hundreds of years, perhaps beginning as early as Chaucer's era in England. The idea of a feast in the middle of month was familiar in ancient Rome, with the Lupercalia festival, which honoured the wolf that suckled Romulus and Remus, as well as being a festival of shepherds and their god Lupercus. It is possible that such mid-month celebrations have eventually become associated with Valentine's Day today.

February should not involve drastic lifestyle changes, but in line with the practices described above, it presents opportunities to start shaking off winter whilst continuing to sustain oneself until the season changes. Buoying up mood and energy levels is important, as for many people, this is a difficult and joyless period. Persevering with a healthier approach for the last part of winter and attending to inner needs will allow greater changes to be made in spring. If winter becomes draining, with reliance on sweets or alcohol, spring will entail repairing the damage, rather than moving forward.

Valentine's day now is mostly a commercial festival – millions of pounds are spent each year on cards, flowers, chocolates and other gifts, and couples dutifully eating overpriced set menus in restaurants is a common sight on February 14. Despite this, it is possible to still celebrate the halfway point of what is generally a dreary month, whether single or part of a couple.

The best supplements for mood and energy

There are many "miracle" supplements for mood and energy, and it is natural to be tempted by the promise of a quick fix, particularly in winter. The following guide focuses on some of the better supplements for mood and energy (see Resources chapter for stockists).

Omega-3 oils

Fish oil provides essential fatty acids (omega-3) that cannot be produced by the body, and which are usually missing from the modern diet. Research has demonstrated the benefits of fish oil supplementation in many situations – it can help improve cardiovascular health (including in at-risk diabetics), reduce arthritic symptoms and help with depression and other mental health disorders. As the types of studies conducted vary significantly – with some being very short, or using low doses of fish oil, there is still an ongoing debate as to the role of fish oil in stabilising mood, although overall it is a well-researched supplement, which is likely to have a beneficial effect on mood, with potential as an adjunctive treatment in some forms of depression and anxiety.

If buying fish oil, choose a brand that states it is free of contaminants such as PCBs (polychlorinated biphenyls), and which gives high levels of EPA and DHA. Generally, doses above 1g per day are required, but check with your GP, especially if you are taking blood thinning medications.

A more recent addition to the omega-3 market is krill oil. There is evidence that the omega-3 oils from krill are better absorbed than those from fish oil, although krill oil is generally less well researched, and more expensive. Additionally, there is an issue with the longer-term sustainability of oils extracted from marine sources, and vegetarian omega-3 oils are available, though these tend to have a less favourable balance of fats, and can quickly become rancid – particularly flax seed oil.

Verdict: Fish oil can be a good investment. It may support

mood, and is likely to have an impact on longer term health. Vegetarian options for omega-3 provision are available.

5-HTP (5- hydroxytryptophan)

Medications that increase brain levels of the neurotransmitter (chemical involved in nerve transmission) serotonin are the first line of therapy for depression. Whilst serotonin deficiency may be a simplistic view, boosting serotonin levels can help with mood and certain forms of depression.

5-HTP supplements are an alternative way increase serotonin levels, as they provide the body with a precursor to the neurotransmitter. Studies have suggested the supplement might have potential in helping improve mood, relaxation and sleep. 5-HTP must not be taken by people using an antidepressant, prescription sleeping pills or St John's wort, and care may also be needed when using certain cold and flu remedies.

Tryptophan, related to 5-HTP, used to be a popular supplement, An outbreak of eosinophilic myalgia, a disabling condition, which can be fatal, was associated with tryptophan supplementation, but this is believed to have been due to contamination of the product during manufacture. Tryptophan is produced industrially, whereas 5-HTP is usually extracted from a plant. 5-HTP is considered to be a safe product, but check for interactions with any supplements or medications before using, and discontinue use and see a healthcare professional if you feel you are developing side effects.

Verdict: Worth considering if low mood, anxiety and poor sleep are a problem. Talk to your doctor too though if you are experiencing any of these symptoms.

B vitamins

B complex vitamins are involved in a wide range of biochemical reactions, and suboptimal levels can lead to feelings of lethargy and low mood. Some experts believe that the current RDA is too low for true good health. Also, certain B vitamins are helpful in reducing levels of homocysteine, a biochemical by-product that is implicated in a number of disease processes, including atherosclerosis and dementia.

Avoiding sub-optimal levels of B vitamins is important, frank deficiency is dangerous, and the importance of folic acid supplementation in pregnancy is well known. B vitamins can be obtained from a wide range of foods, including meat and whole grains, but trying a good quality B complex may be warranted for lethargy. Vegetarians often need to supplement with vitamin B12 as this is not as easily obtained from non-animal sources.

High doses of B6 can lead to nerve damage, and so care is required if using a high-dose B complex product.

Verdict: Avoid deficiency, and consider a supplement if lethargy is a problem.

Magnesium

This is a mineral involved in many important biochemical reactions. Deficiency can be caused by intense exercise, stress and dietary factors, and can bring about a range of symptoms and predispositions to disease, including potentially anxiety, disturbed sleep and PMS

Verdict: Correcting a magnesium deficiency may help with energy levels and general wellbeing, although accurate testing of magnesium levels may be difficult and costly. Where lethargy is a problem, trying a good quality magnesium chelate supplement may be the easiest course of action, that also represents the best value for money.

L-carnitine

This amino acid based supplement may improve the function of the insulin system, protect against oxidative stress and support brain function, although results of studies are not conclusive. Deficiency of carnitine can prevent effective fat burning, as the molecule is required for the transportation of fat into mitochondria (the part of the cell where fat is used to create energy) and correcting such a deficiency should – in theory – help with fat loss. Anecdotal evidence suggests that l-carnitine supplements can be useful for fat loss and for improving alertness.

Verdict: Can be bought cheaply, so may be worth a try if you require an alertness boost, and are also interested in breaking a fat loss plateau.

Is it the time of year, or is it something else?

Many people feel less energetic during the darker months, and identifying and correcting a nutritional deficiency, and maintaining a balance between rest and physical activity, can be helpful in restoring vitality. Where tiredness and lethargy have become significant features of life for some time though, it may be worth considering other possibilities.

See how many of the following statements apply to you:

Do you feel tired all the time, no matter how much sleep you get?

Is getting out of bed in the morning a difficult, drawn out process, no matter how you feel about the upcoming day?

Do you rely on caffeine and/or sweet foods to get through the day?

Do you sometimes feel tired during the day but anxious and unable to fall asleep at night?

Does your mind feel permanently "foggy", and are you more forgetful than you used to be?

Is it difficult to remember the last time you felt energetic and full of life?

Do you have a very stressful lifestyle, or did you have a stressful lifestyle in the past?

Have you had hair loss, dry skin, digestive or menstrual disturbances?
Do you sometimes feel dizzy if you stand up too quickly?
If you are female, do you have very heavy periods?

If you identify with one or more of the above, you may be suffering from a thyroid and/or adrenal imbalance, or you may be anaemic.

Thyroid disorders

The thyroid gland is situated in the neck and releases hormones that control metabolism. Disorders of the gland often have an autoimmune cause (the immune system attacks the body's own cells). The symptoms of an overactive thyroid include weight loss, usually despite an increased appetite, anxiety and a rapid heartbeat. Thyroid under-activity is more common, and causes weight gain, lethargy, depression and hair loss, amongst other symptoms.

GPs will usually test for an underactive thyroid when a patient complains of persistent tiredness, and in some cases a thyroid disease is diagnosed, and treatment is prescribed. However, there are many of people who experience low thyroid-type symptoms, and have blood test results that are a little high or low, but which do not correspond with what is deemed "abnormal". These people can be considered to have a "subclinical" thyroid problem.

The tests comprising a thyroid function panel include thyroid stimulating hormone (TSH), thyroxine (T4) and T3, the short acting form of thyroxine. TSH is a hormone released by the pituitary gland that signals to the thyroid gland to release its hormones, which control metabolism. As with many other body systems, this is controlled by a feedback loop – thyroid hormones suppress TSH release, meaning that the levels of circulating hormones should remain within specific levels. If the thyroid produces a large amount of thyroid hormone, or thyroid hormones are introduced into the body, TSH is strongly suppressed, and may become undetectable. When the thyroid is sluggish, more TSH is produced, in an effort to stimulate the thyroid to increase its output.

Some experts believe that the "normal range" for TSH, which varies between laboratories, is generally too broad. Depending on the laboratory, a TSH of up to 5 mU/L may be normal, although some doctors feel that any value above 2mU/L represent a sluggish thyroid. The issue is that GPs and many specialists would consider such levels to be normal.

There are further issues with the blood tests used – T3 is not always routinely tested. It is possible to have normal levels of TSH and thyroxine, but if there is a problem with the conversion of thyroxine to T3,hypothyroid symptoms can result, since T3 is the main short-term effector of the thyroid. Additionally, the free forms of the thyroid hormones should be assessed – the hormones circulate bound to a protein, where they are unable to act. So it is possible to have normal "total" levels, but an insufficient proportion of hormones available to act.

Finally, even when a thyroid problem is diagnosed, treatment tends to be with thyroxine alone – just one of the hormones that the thyroid produces. Some people, when supplied with extra thyroxine, can produce the remaining thyroid hormones from it, but this is not always the case.

What to do:

- Ask for a blood test and request your blood test results. If you suspect you may fall into the subclinical category, there is action you can take to help yourself. Start with cleaning up your diet, and ensuring you have an adequate intake of proteins and trace elements (required by the thyroid). You might also want to seek the advice of an alternative health practitioner, and try out thyroid

support formulae, such as Nutri thyroid (glandular, hormone free)
- Supporting the adrenals is sometimes required to boost thyroid function (see below)
- If you are taking thyroxine but still experiencing low thyroid symptoms, request a free T3 test. Also try discussing natural thyroid with your doctor – this is an animal sourced product which provides all the hormones and co factors usually made by the thyroid. Formulations are usually from pigs, so may not be suitable for everyone

Adrenal fatigue

Adrenal fatigue has been named the "21st century disorder", but it is still largely unrecognised by the medical profession. The adrenals are small glands situated above the kidneys, responsible for secreting, among others, the "fight or flight" hormones adrenaline and cortisol. These hormones prepare the body for action, by raising heartbeat and alertness, dilating the pupils, ensuring blood sugar levels are adequate and temporarily shutting down processes that are not immediately relevant to survival, such as digestion.

The adrenals are designed to be stimulated occasionally, for short periods – for example, when escaping from a predator or fighting for a precious resource. In the modern setting, they are stimulated on a daily basis, by everyday stressors, which the body's systems cannot recognise as being minor in terms of survival. This situation can have longer term negative impacts on health through cortisol excess, and ultimately, through the adrenals becoming "over-worked". A particularly strong case of flu or pneumonia, or an operation, can also adversely affect adrenal function.

The key symptoms of adrenal fatigue include very low morning energy and strong reliance on caffeine and sugar to "get through the day". Sufferers may find they have more energy in the evenings, finding it difficult to relax and sleep, compounding the problem. This is due to an unbalanced cortisol rhythm (see August chapter for more on cortisol) – normally levels of cortisol are higher in the morning, and decrease throughout the day, tailing off in the evening, preparing the body for sleep. Where the adrenals are fatigued, the glands only start producing enough cortisol to cause physiological arousal towards evening – the subsequent poor sleep preventing any regeneration. As adrenal fatigue progresses, a sufferer may move from feeling "tired but wired", to simply exhausted, corresponding to a flat cortisol rhythm.

What to do:

- Saliva tests from private labs are perhaps the most reliable tests for adrenal fatigue (the usual blood tests are often of little help), but this can be expensive, so it may be worth discussing a trial of adrenal support with an integrative health practitioner, if the symptoms fit. Start by reviewing your diet. Whilst it is not necessary to cut out caffeine or sweet treats entirely, avoid relying on them for energy
- Consider a good quality vitamin and mineral supplement including B vitamins and vitamin C. Ask about glandular, hormone free formulae for adrenal support
- Make an effort to reset your cortisol rhythm. Active relaxation in the evening, and supplements such as phosphatidylserine can help to decrease cortisol levels and promote sleep
- Listen to your body. When you feel you need to rest – do so wherever possible. Plan in recuperation and modify activities such as exercise in accordance with other aspects of your schedule. For example, if a particularly long working day is on the horizon, avoiding tiring activities such as heavy exercise beforehand. After a demanding exercise session, make sure you recover adequately

Anaemia

Common in women due to menstrual blood loss, anaemia can be responsible for tiredness and lethargy. Haemoglobin level is usually one of the first tests requested by a doctor when a patient presents with tiredness, but to fully understand the body's iron balance, it is necessary to look at other parts of the iron system, such as ferritin. Generally, haemoglobin is the last part of the system to change and low levels indicate that iron stores are somewhat depleted.

Low levels of ferritin can be cause hair loss, and supplementing with iron can prevent further loss.

What to do:

- Ask your doctor to test for ferritin as well as haemoglobin
- If you are anaemic, discuss the range of iron supplements available with your GP. Those usually prescribed can be harsh and constipating, and may be poorly absorbed. Natural forms of iron, such as those found in formulations such as Floradix or Spatone, may be better absorbed and have fewer side effects
- Take iron with vitamin C to increase absorption
- Increase sources of iron in your diet. This is more difficult for vegetarians, but it is still possible to include foods such as spinach, apricots and pumpkin seeds, which are rich in the mineral. For non-vegetarians, good quality red meat is an excellent source of iron. Health concerns over red meat relate largely to poor quality processed meats, such as sausages and ham. Good quality meat, from grass-fed, organically raised animals is a nutritious, healthy choice

Ways to boost health, wellbeing and mood in February

Food and drink

Eating correctly can improve energy levels and support the immune system, but meals should be interesting and enjoyable as well as healthy. Vegetables are commonly thought of as the nutritious, but boring part of meals, but cooking them in interesting ways needn't be complicated. The following websites can provide a starting point for creating delicious vegetable dishes:

http://www.jamieoliver.com/recipes/
http://www.bbc.co.uk/food/
http://www.waitrose.com/food/cookingandrecipes/index.aspx

Many people rely more heavily on caffeine during winter, and it is not necessary cut out tea and coffee. Consider swapping some cups of coffee for green tea and try to cut out caffeine after 4pm, as when consumed later in the day it can disturb sleep, reinforcing the cycle of daytime lethargy and requirement for caffeine.

Exercise

Brisk walks on bright winter days can be invigorating, although in the UK damp, grey days prevail, meaning that indoor exercise is likely to be preferred . For those with an established exercise routine, consider adding variety with exercise classes, or ask for advice from a personal trainer or fitness instructor to create a routine that can be performed in parallel to the existing one – if the focus of an existing programme is on resistance work, spend some days on flexibility, for example.

If you do not yet have an exercise routine, see the January chapter for ideas on increasing activity levels without a gym. Being more active is one way to combat the dullness of the early part of the year.

Pampering and relaxation

Evoke the purifying and warming energies of fire – invest in some attractive scented candles, or better still, look for candle-making courses or kits and create your own.

Check local spas for special offers (see Resources section for discount websites), or enjoy a spa experience at home with luxury bathing products. Look out for steam room and sauna facilities at local leisure centres, where prices are significantly lower than spas.

Winter evenings are perfect for becoming engrossed in a book – joining a local library is free, and may also raise your awareness of community events. Reading is relaxing as it allows attention to be shifted entirely from everyday stresses, and may be preferable to television as a method of winding down for those who work in front of a screen during the day.

Celebrate the middle of the month – why not mark the halfway point of February with a lovingly prepared meal or an enjoyable activity – this does not have to be aligned to the commercial interests around Valentine's day. See the next section for ideas.

Aphrodisiac meals – fact and fiction

Certain foods have become part of Valentine's day meals as aphrodisiacs, although there is little evidence that any food can increase sexual desire or performance in humans.

Seafood, particularly oysters, is widely thought to have aphrodisiac properties – the high zinc content (needed for production of sperm in males) is thought to be responsible, although a high zinc meal is unlikely to have immediate effect. Care must be taken with seafood, particularly in restaurants, because of the possibility of food-borne illness – the highly contagious norovirus can be contracted from eating shellfish.

Other foods reputed to be aphrodisiacs, such as asparagus, most likely gained their reputation because of their shape, texture, etc. The lack of evidence for aphrodisiac foods does not mean that creating a romantic meal, which could heighten feelings of desire or bring about a relaxed mood, is not possible though.

Firstly, avoid foods that you or your potential lover may have unfavourable reactions to – these can be as common as wheat and dairy, which can cause bloating and digestive disturbances – not conducive to romance. Also avoid very strong flavours and overly-spiced dishes. Keep the meal fairly light as feelings of over-fullness leads to lethargy and discomfort. Stimulate the senses with a range of textures and colours, and also harmonise flavours, avoiding being too adventurous and introducing discordance. Part of feeling relaxed and resonsive to another person is feeling comfortable with yourself, so carefully consider the use of messy foods that are difficult to eat elegantly (e.g., spaghetti), whilst keeping in mind the sensory aspect of using fingers to eat (e.g., vegetables and dips).

Sweet foods can provide a temporary serotonin boost, and are associated with indulgence and sensuality, so a dessert can be important at a romantic meal. Don't choose something overly sweet, as this is likely to lead to an energy dip shortly after eating, due to a sharp spike of insulin. Instead, balance out flavours and textures. The mood-enhancing effects of chocolate may be more anecdotal than evidence-based, but if you or your partner enjoys it, it is worth including on the romantic menu.

Small amounts of alcohol can reduce feelings of inhibition, but take care not over-consume. Avoiding fizzy drinks may be a good idea, as these can cause digestive discomfort. Finish off the meal with a herbal tea, such as ginger, peppermint or fennel to aid digestion.

Chapter summary

- February is a time of looking forward towards spring, and of completing the winter season
- This month, consider how to boost mood and energy levels

through nutrition, supplements and lifestyle changes

- Nature is stirring, and warmer days are approaching – ensure your body is appropriately supported, and ready for the change; resist the temptation to get through the remaining dark days with sugar, caffeine or alcohol

Workbook section

Winter reflections

How I felt this winter:

Energy levels

Mood

Winter-specific habits that were helpful(e.g, spending more time with family, taking longer over cooking), and unhelpful (e.g., too much chocolate and red wine in the evenings):

How I would like next winter to be different:

February

How I usually feel in February:

What would I like to change this year:

Signs I have seen that spring is approaching:

How I am removing associations to winter in my life:

March

Make a change!

March is usually cold and blustery, and can often feel like winter, but it is a time of change. New buds and blossoms are starting to be visible, and the vernal equinox at the end of the month marks equality between day and night. In Anglo-Saxon lore, March (Hrethmonath) was associated with the war goddess Hretha and with notions of winter being conquered.

There are yet more connections with battle – in English, the name of the month comes from the Roman god of war, Mars. From the Chinese perspective, the energy of spring is the somewhat aggressive energy of growing wood, which directs itself upwards, out of the earth. March is ideal for a campaign of your own. Many people find their energy levels begin to increase once the days start to lengthen – this extends to sexual interest too, mirrored in the animal world by the start of the mating season for many species.

Despite nature's new starts, it is also quite common to encounter spring tiredness in March – a temporary form of fatigue and lethargy, thought to be due to the body taking time to adjust to the surge of hormones and neurotransmitters caused by the increasing levels of light. It is therefore important not to overdo any new diet or exercise regimes.

The capricious nature of the month is underlined in the Bulgarian ritual of Martenitsa – on the first day of March, Bulgarians exchange and wear white and red tassels to gain the favour of the grumpy Baba Marta (old woman March) and allow spring to arrive earlier. A wearer can remove the tassels once they see signs of spring, such as a stork or a tree in blossom – the tassels are then hung on a tree.

Whilst Easter may sometimes fall in March, often much of the month is taken up with the period of Lent, and so typically there were few opportunities for public celebration. Exceptions are the Annunciation (25 March), which for several centuries marked the New Year in England, the feasts of Irish and Welsh saints and Mothers' Day. The origins of this last festival may be largely practical. By the middle of Lent, winter food stores would be running low, and so older female family members may have required assistance. Eventually, Mothers' Day became mostly an opportunity for domestic servants and apprentices to visit their families, and almost disappeared in the early 20th century, before being revived in the US and then the UK.

Lent is preceded by the opportunity to use up foods not permitted during the period of abstinence (Shrove Tuesday, Pancake Day), and in the past Shrovetide involved a variety of public events. In some countries, carnivals are still held before Lent begins, providing an opportunity to have fun before a particularly sombre period begins.

Whilst March may not fully feel like spring, increased energy levels and the noticeable lengthening of the days mean it is the ideal month to make diet and lifestyle changes. From a practical perspective, making significant changes in March means there is sufficient time to feel and see a difference by summer, and to form habits before the distractions of the warmer weather.

Spring – time for a cleanse?

Fasting and abstinence during early springtime are familiar to Christians because of the austerity of Lent. As well as having religious implications, a period of restriction in early spring may have fitted well with the agrarian calendar – stores of food and fuel would have been low after the winter, and it would have been a time of increased activity in terms of ploughing and sowing, meaning little opportunity for feasting.

The idea of marking the new season with a change of eating habits that may also stimulate changes can be appealing, but dramatic changes do not suit everyone.

Detox

There is significant debate over the term "detox". Modern environments, particularly in cities, are loaded with potentially harmful chemicals, and the problems caused by poisoning with lead, mercury and organic compounds are well known. There is evidence that as well as causing immediate poisoning, certain chemicals , such as those found in pesticides, can cause longer term damage where exposure is low-grade.

Whilst true allergy to "chemicals" is quite rare, a significant number of people are sensitive to even commonplace products, such as household cleaning aids, air fresheners and soaps, and the sensitivity can manifest as headaches, rashes and digestive disturbances when exposure occurs. In the last century, a bewildering array of chemical compounds has entered the environment, and we are also exposed to a greater level of "natural" but potentially harmful substances too, such as heavy metals. It is therefore no surprise that specialised "detox" regimes and supplements are popular – they are thought to reduce the "toxic load" on the body, enhancing health and fat loss.

Whilst removing an offending chemical from a person's environment can have immediate and longer term beneficial effects, and common sense would lead us to assume that reducing exposure to compounds and metals that can adversely affect the body's systems might be helpful, the term "detox" is much overused. The body has its own "detox" systems – enzymes in the liver, which modify both internally produced and external chemicals, rendering them inactive. It is possible for these systems to become overloaded, but this is only medically recognised in the case of acute poisoning, e.g., by paracetamol. Supporting the liver enzymes with good nutrition, specific phytochemicals and trace elements may be beneficial, but care must be taken around many of the expensive and complicated "detox" products and services – many of these may be no more than prettily packaged multivitamins, fibre supplements or sweating treatments.

True "detox" by its very nature should be simple, involving a reduction in the amount of stimuli that the body has to process, and can be achieved through the following:

- Eating mostly unprocessed organic foods. Whilst organic foods are generally superior in terms of being produced with fewer human interferences, ensuring food is not refined or processed is also important – a sweet organic snack is better than a chocolate bar containing additives and trans-fats, but high levels of sugar (even organic sugar, or fructose) will stress the body
- Drinking plenty of good quality water. Ideally mineral water from a glass bottle, or filtered tap water. Water straight from the tap can contain high levels of unwanted substances
- Exercise. Human bodies were designed to be active and exercise stimulates lymphatic flow, important for the elimination of wastes from the tissues
- Access to fresh air. Recycled or polluted air can contribute to allergies, and to feelings of lethargy. Making time to breathe cleaner air can boost energy

Fasting

Fasting can be considered an extreme form of "detox" - it eliminates stress on the body from food and drink, and requires the body to use its own energy stores as fuel.

Fasting has been used for centuries, and some people find it helps boost fat loss, as well as improving mental clarity. Others find fasting has a negative impact on metabolism, particularly if they have a sluggish thyroid – or that it is simply unpleasant and impractical with no benefits.

If you are considering a fast for the first time, it may be worth trying it in a quiet period, for example over a long weekend, or when on holiday (although take care if in a warmer climate), and under supervision. Check with your doctor that fasting is safe for you, and keep fasts short, unless under close supervision. When fat is used as energy, substances stored in the fat may be released, therefore it is important to drink plenty of water throughout.

Some forms of fast involve eating only one type of food, and this may be a better approach than fasting on liquids alone for those new to the approach.

Raw foods and juices

Again, responses to regimes involving raw foods and juices are highly variable. Some may feel energised by a juicing regime, others who are sensitive to fruit sugar may actually gain fat and another group may see no difference apart from lethargy and upset digestion.

As cooking decreases the nutrient content of foods, and also makes it easier to digest, it makes sense not to overcook vegetables, for example. A lightly steamed serving of carrots retains more of the beneficial phytochemicals, and may keep you fuller than overcooked mush. Taking this further, some people feel much better on a diet of largely raw foods.

A measure of trial and error may be required in determining whether raw foods or juices will be useful for an individual. Keep in mind that in many cultures, cold foods are avoided during cold weather, as it is believed that consuming cold food or drink in the wrong situations can bring on illness, and also that cold foods and drinks should be avoided when ill. Additionally, very cold foods and drinks may not be helpful in hot weather – witness the use of warm mint teas in Middle Eastern countries to promote cooling, as the body reacts to the warm liquid by decreasing its temperature.

There may not be scientific support for the beliefs about cold foods and cold environments, but they do appeal to common sense. A week of juicing or raw food in relaxed, warm surroundings may have a very different impact to trying to integrate these methods into a busy life in a city in a temperate zone. Whilst eating more raw or lightly cooked vegetables may be beneficial for everyone, a diet consisting solely of these is unlikely to suit the majority of people living in colder climates.

Other ideas for kickstarts

For a kickstart with less divergence from everyday life, a period of discipline, similar to the introductory phases of the Dukan Diet or Atkins Diet may be helpful, as long as this is safe for you. Focus on good quality proteins, vegetables (cooked or raw), avoiding all processed food and most grains. If you prefer to include a complex carbohydrate, include brown rice.

Also commit to drinking more good quality water during this period, and to moving more.

A new plan for spring

Whether or not the season starts with a "detox", or a period of disciplined eating, if fat loss or greater energy is the goal, early spring is the time to make diet and lifestyle changes. The following are some ideas for progressing with a wellbeing boosting or fat loss plan.

Examine your relationship with the sweet taste

Perhaps at the start of the year, you started to cut down on superfluous sweet snacks, such as sugary mid morning boosts and habits such as a coffee and a muffin. Now be more critical about your relationship with the sweet taste. Have you cut down on desserts, but replaced them with supposedly "healthy" flapjacks, protein bars or diet drinks, or increased your fruit intake? If so, it is likely that you are still craving the sweet taste, and may be sabotaging any efforts to lose fat or improve your lifestyle through including sweet-tasting foods too often.

What to do:

- Consider 2 weeks without any sweet tasting food or refined carbohydrate (white bread, pasta, white rice). One cause of sweet/carbohydrate cravings is high levels of insulin – caused by eating sweets and refined carbohydrates. Reducing insulin levels will remove the "physiological" aspect of the craving
- If this seems too strict, try removing sweet tasting foods from your diet 6 days per week, and allowing yourself one or two meals to really enjoy genuine sweet foods – not replacements. This approach might be difficult if you have an "all or nothing" approach to nutrition though
- Supplements such as magnesium, 5-HTP (see February chapter) and chromium may be useful in reducing cravings. One aspect of chocolate craving may involve magnesium deficiency, and self-medication with serotonin-boosting sweets is common in people with low mood
- Take care with fruit intake. Whilst generally considered to be healthy, fruit contains high levels of sugar (fructose), as do natural sweeteners such as honey and agave nectar. Fructose has little impact on insulin (low insulin index), but if it is not required immediately for energy or re-fuelling, it is processed in the liver and stored as fat. The best fruits are fibrous and/or less sweet, such as apples, cherries and berries. Considering the seasonality of fruit, which has now been lost, it is a food that would only have been available usually only in late summer and autumn. This could be considered a period where it would have been beneficial to cool down with fresh-tasting foods, and to begin to store fat, in readiness for the colder months. Regularly eating sweet tropical fruits, and especially juices or smoothies, can for some people, bring fat loss to a halt

- Finally, simply identifying where sweet eating is just a habit or an activity to bring comfort or relieve boredom can be helpful. Replace the sweet snack with another food or activity

Review your carbohydrate intake

Protein, fat and carbohydrate are the three macronutrients. Protein and fat have synthetic roles in the body – protein is used in building muscle and bone and in the synthesis of neurotransmitters. Cell membranes are made of fats, and hormones are based on fats. The only role of carbohydrate is to provide energy.

Viewed in this way, it is clear that carbohydrates are not "the enemy", and also why restricting them can help with fat loss. Carbohydrates can be essential for those who are physically active, particularly people with smaller stores of energy as fat. For those looking to lose fat and who are not physically active, starchy, concentrated carbohydrates may be somewhat unnecessary, and will prevent fat loss – seeing as it is easier for ingested carbohydrate to be used as fuel for most activities, than for fat to be mobilised.

The role of starches is often too central in our society. Pasta, which in Italy is typically a prelude to the main course, is commonly thought of as a meal in itself in the UK. Basing meals on carbohydrate may have been necessary for the survival of poorer agrarian people in the past, as a large amount of cheap "fuel" was required for day after day of physical labour. Unless you engage in hard physical work or intensive exercise on a regular basis, carbohydrate should be an accompaniment to a meal, with the focus being on vegetables and protein.

What to do

- It is not necessary to cut out carbohydrates completely, but do work towards cutting out refined and processed versions – white bread and sandwiches, commercial snacks and sweets, white pasta and all forms of "junk food". Brown rice, quinoa, oats, legumes and root vegetable are all more complex forms of carbohydrate, which can be enjoyed by people on fat loss plans

- Make starchy carbohydrates a smaller part of your meals, and avoid having carbohydrate based meals, unless you are very physically active. Also consider avoiding starchy carbohydrates entirely on days when you are neither physically active nor recovering from intense exercise

Review your use of dairy products

It is wise to reconsider your use of dairy – using small amounts as a condiment can help to maintain variety in the diet, but large, regular amounts may be better avoided.

Firstly, some trial and error may be required to determine whether you are able to tolerate dairy at all. The incidence of lactose intolerance varies widely across ethnic groups, and there can be a dose-response effect with dairy products, fluctuating tolerance levels, or the ability to tolerate some dairy products, but not others.

Lactose intolerance is due to low levels or absence of lactase, the intestinal enzyme which breaks down the milk sugar lactose. In the absence of the enzyme, lactose is fermented by intestinal bacteria, leading to the discomfort, bloating, wind and diarrhoea associated with lactose intolerance. Lactose intolerance is relatively rare in people of northern European heritage, but more frequent in southern Europeans, and is almost universal in some Asian groups. It is not lactose alone in dairy products that can cause problems – it is possible to be sensitive to milk proteins, and some people find they cope much better with goat's milk as opposed to cow's milk, even though goat's milk also contains lactose. There are now a variety of milk substitute products available, such as oat, rice hemp and nut "milks."

The high calcium content of dairy is thought to be responsible for its beneficial effects on bone health, and its ability to support fat loss, although vitamin D3 may be more important for bone health than calcium.

Regarding fat loss, dairy products are unusual in that there is a mismatch between their impact on blood sugar (low) and the response of insulin (high) – excessive stimulation of insulin means that dairy products can encourage fat storage. On the other hand, as dairy products can be quite satisfying and enjoyable, a small portion of hard cheese or a yogurt could replace an unhealthy snack such as crisps or a chocolate bar, and making such choices could lead to fat loss.

There are particular areas of concern for women regarding dairy intake – high intakes of low fat dairy products have been linked to anovulatory infertility (although high fat intake from dairy had the opposite effect). Some studies report reduced breast cancer risk in women who regularly eat dairy – perhaps due to vitamin D - whilst other researchers propose a connection between the hormones and growth promoters in milk and breast cancer, and low levels of dairy consumption are another potential reason for lower breast cancer rates in Japan.

Finally, decreasing dairy consumption can be helpful for people with respiratory problems and allergies such as hayfever; many people find that cutting out dairy decreases mucus congestion.

What to do

- If you can tolerate dairy products, and enjoy them, it is not necessary to cut them out completely, unless you are particularly concerned about potential impacts on your health. Limiting use is advisable for everyone. View dairy products as a condiment to be used to add interest to meals and prevent boredom, not as a part of your daily diet. Avoid drinking large quantities of milk or using milk on cereals

- Always choose the best quality products available, and the most natural forms, organic where possible. Choose full fat over reduced fat, as low fat dairy products are more processed and often have added sugar, plus altering the fat profile of dairy products has poorly understood and potentially harmful effects on the body
- If you need to replace dairy products, do not be tempted to use soy milk or yogurt, as soy can have adverse effects on the thyroid and other hormones. There is a wide variety of milk substitutes available – nut milk, oat milk, hemp milk, quinoa milk, and it is possible to make many of these at home
- If you are concerned about bone health, speak to your doctor, but also make sure you have an adequate intake of vitamin D (see October chapter). Regular weight-bearing exercise can also be helpful for keeping bones and joints strong and functional

Exercise

Commit to being more active and exercising more. Whilst these points are linked, there is an important difference – being more active involves walking instead of using transport and making other opportunities to move the body. Exercising, or better still "training", involves progressive effort, with the idea of making changes to the physical state.

Increasing activity in early spring is in line with the changes in the natural world. Lengthening days and the appearance of milder weather means people as well as animals are enticed from their cocoons of winter sleepiness.

How to approach exercise

For an exercise plan to work and to be feasible in the long term, it should be tailored to an individual's physical, and psychological needs. Consider the following:

- Do you enjoy having a routine, and find it easy to follow plans consistently, working towards goals when these have been set?
- Are you easily bored, generally more interested in mental, rather than physical pursuits and need a "reason" to exercise?
- Do you exercise out of compulsion, to release mental energy or relieve stress, and do you find that your exercise behaviour tends to be erratic?

Those that respond well to routine and clear goals can achieve excellent results with regular exercise, as they remain committed and stick to their plans. The key for individuals of this type is avoiding being "stuck in a rut", following a routine out of habit, whether that is attending the same exercise classes, or using one gym programme for 6 months. Regular review, with updates as necessary, sub-goals and check points will help this type of person put their staying power to the best use.

People requiring an intellectual reason to exercise and who are easily bored may need a different approach – setting goals may not make much difference in the long term, unless these have a specific type of meaning for the individual. For example, whilst people of this type may understand the benefits of reaching a certain weight/body fat level, unless working towards and achieving this goal has durable intellectual appeal, boredom will set in and the plan will be abandoned. As well as identifying a true reason to exercise, variety may also be important, so people of this type would not respond as well to having a fixed routine with clear sub-goals and checkpoints.

People who exercise out of compulsion, or for psychological reasons may also respond less well in the long term to goals – these can be achieved, and then discarded, or there may be a large discrepancy between "on plan" and "off plan" behaviour (all or nothing). In these instances, an exercise routine should be balanced, perhaps including techniques such as yoga, as well as some aspect of a regular routine to provide a measure of security. A mixture of high intensity and lower intensity work will prevent fixation on a particular form of activity. Additionally, other aspects of the person's life should also be examined, and the psychological issues addressed where possible.

Which type of exercise?

For those looking to make changes to their shape or body fat level, resistance exercise, coupled with changes to the diet and perhaps interval cardiovascular training is the best way to achieve goals. The stress on the muscles during a weights workout means that post-exercise repair is required. To carry out this repair, the body uses fat as fuel. Simply having a greater percentage of lean mass (more muscle compared to fat) means an enhanced metabolic rate and the ability to use more calories at rest.

Resistance work is also the only way to achieve a shapely look, but many women avoid it for fear of developing a masculine physique. This is compounded by the ineffective "women's exercises" often prescribed by fitness professionals, and perhaps by some of the pervasive ideas about femininity – women are conditioned to believe that being physically strong is the domain of men, and also that sweating and lifting weights is unattractive. In addition to being the most effective route to changing body shape, weight bearing exercise is also key in preventing osteoporosis, and so should be a part of a woman's exercise regime.

Women build muscle at the same rate as men, but female muscles are smaller – and so whilst a woman will see an increase in muscle mass, it would be extremely difficult for her to build the same type of muscle mass as a man, or to look "male", without using androgens ("male" hormones, anabolic steroids). It is also possible to adapt a resistance training programme to deliver increases in strength, without large changes in muscle size.

As women naturally have more subcutaneous body fat than men, increases in muscle size can lead to a bulky, rather than a defined look, when body fat levels are maintained. The resistance training itself will help to reduce body fat, but it is also important to pay attention to the diet, if you want to create a lean look – in particular being careful not to over-eat calorie dense foods. Resistance work can be exhausting, and the mistake of over-eating the wrong foods after sessions, or reducing activity too much on non-training days is quite common.

See the January chapter for practical ideas on getting started with exercise without a gym, and the Resources section for information on choosing a gym and a Personal Trainer.

Spring tiredness

Spring tiredness is thought to be due to increasing levels of hormones and neurotransmitters putting a strain on the body. A period of lethargy in early springtime can be addressed through the following:

- Identifying where a more complex problem may be involved (see February Chapter for information on thyroid and adrenal imbalances)
- Resting when a cold or similar minor illness is beginning – trying to "work through" an infection can lead to weeks of feeling sub-par
- Good sleep habits (see April Chapter)
- Good nutrition
- Regular exercise, in harmony with energy levels. Moderate exercise can often provide a boost, but reserve more intense sessions for when you have more energy
- Not allowing occasional "slips" in the diet – such as sugary foods eaten to provide an energy burst – to derail a healthy eating plan. If such slips occur, then they should be accepted, and not dwelt on

Chapter summary

- March may still feel like winter, but it is the time to make changes to diet and lifestyle. Re-examine your relationship with the sweet taste -avoiding sweets and refined carbohydrates for a while can help to reduce cravings
- Also review your intake of starchy carbohydrates generally, and of dairy products. Dairy products can be connected with allergies and other health problems, and may contribute to fat gain
- Harmonise with the season and become more active; where possible, start a focused training programme

Workbook section

Associations March usually has for me:

Signs of the new season that I have noticed:

Why I think this might be a good time to make changes to my lifestyle:

General changes I hope to make in the coming months:

Changes to my diet I will make this month:

Changes to my activity levels/training regime I will make this month:

April

Renewal and new opportunities

April begins, in the capricious character of early spring, with April fool's day, an institution for several centuries in England. As the month where Easter is often celebrated though, it is a period of new life and renewal.

The English name of the month may correspond to the Latin aprire, to open, as buds are opening now. The month was associated with the goddess Venus, with her festival being held on the first day, and another possibility is that its name derives from her Greek equivalent, Aphrodite. In the Slavic languages that do not use the Latin month names, the name of the month reflects the changes in nature, for example – duben (Czech, oak month – when leaves appear on larger trees), kviten', kwiecien (Ukrainian, Polish – flower month), travanj (Croatian – grass month), krasavik (Belarusian – month of beauty).

In many European countries, the name of the Easter festival is based on the Latin pascha, which is in turn derived from the Hebrew pesach (Passover), but the English term comes from the Germanic. St Bede described a spring or dawn goddess, Ostara/Eostre, whose festival had been celebrated by the pagan peoples in England during Ostarmonath, equivalent to April – although his are the only accounts referring to such a goddess. Whatever the origins of the name of the feast, it has been a great celebration for centuries, mirroring the joyous mood of nature. Hocktide was the period after Easter given over to recreation, and as with Shrovetide before Lent, public celebration could often become riotous or violent.

Rabbits and hares are symbols of Easter, perhaps because of their fertility. Eggs, with their promise of new life, are also part of Easter; traditionally they were forbidden during Lent. The concept of the Easter bunny bringing eggs may be a combination of these two concepts, a reference to the super-fertility of hares, or it may have grown from a legend of an egg-laying hare – unlike rabbits, hares have nests, which may have been confused with birds' nests.

Pre-Christian springtime renewal celebrations were observed in ancient Rome, with the Hilaria festival in honour of the mother goddess Cybele, a Phrygian deity.

This is clearly a time for renewal, as well as for considering new opportunities and the blossoming of ideas. Build on any new starts made in March, and "spring clean" habits and attitudes towards healthy living and fat loss.

Enjoying Easter - healthily

Easter has always been an occasion for joy, and an Easter holiday, with rest from labour, has been a custom for hundreds of years. In terms of health and wellbeing, particularly if spring was started with a period of greater discipline with diet and lifestyle, Easter is an ideal opportunity to relax and indulge in favourite dishes.

Easter food customs include hot cross buns, which may have originated from the belief that foods baked on good Friday had protective powers, and eggs. Throughout the ages, eggs have been both eaten and used as decoration or as part of a game at Easter.

Today in the UK, the Easter holiday tends to involve overindulgence on chocolate eggs and alcohol, and reliance on convenience food. Whilst relaxing now is natural and beneficial, a binge may be sufficient to derail healthy living initiatives for several weeks, and for those with an "all or nothing" mentality, it may herald the end of a plan entirely. Whilst our forbears would have indulged as much as possible in food and drink over the Easter holidays, most work done in the past was physical in nature, and so a week of feasting would have provided energy for upcoming labour in the fields; additionally, whilst refined sugar and flour have been widely available since the 19th century, many of the foods making up the modern diet, and their harmful effects, did not exist until relatively recently.

Answer the following questions to see if your Easter holidays could be re-focused:

- I often go away for Easter, or visit family, which means I have less control over what I eat and how I spend my time
- I like to completely relax at Easter and, as I want a few days' break from thinking about food, I tend to end up relying on ready meals
- I have plenty of chocolate at Easter
- I tend to drink lots of alcohol at Easter
- I don't usually find time to be active at Easter

If you have answered "yes" to any of the above, it may be worth considering a few simple ways to enjoy the Easter holidays in a healthier way:

- Plan ahead – where possible, ensure that you have adequate stocks of easy to prepare, healthy foods for the Easter holiday, to prevent reliance on convenience foods. This could include frozen portions of home-cooked meals
- If spending Easter abroad, or visiting family or friends, you will have less control over what you eat. When you can, make the healthier choice (e.g., when eating out, choose grilled fish, poultry and meat with vegetables or salad over large pasta dishes), and avoid foods such as crisps or chocolate, eaten just out of habit – snack on nuts or lower GI fruits such as apples and berries during the day to keep hunger at bay, and try to start the day with a protein-based breakfast.
- It is not necessary to cut out alcohol over Easter, but cutting down will help you stay focused on a healthier

lifestyle – you will feel more clear headed, make better food choices and not have to deal with the metabolic negatives of alcohol

- Consider the plans for any children you may be spending the Easter holiday with. Adults often end up overindulging on chocolate, as a result of the chocolate eggs given to children, so it may be worth giving alternative presents, which will benefit all involved. Active Easter games could also be worth introducing, including an Easter Egg hunt (the eggs in question could be painted hen's eggs, instead of chocolate eggs)

Sleep

With the focus on renewal in April, it is fitting to consider the importance of healthy sleep, as it is during sleep that many bodily renewal processes can take place.

Answer the following questions to help determine if your sleep is optimal.

- Do you get less sleep than you need most nights of the week?
- Do you awake feeling unrefreshed?
- Is your sleep often interrupted, e.g., by trips to the toilet, a partner's snoring, or the presence of pets?
- Do you keep electrical equipment in your bedroom?
- Do you use your bedroom for activities other than sleep and sex?
- Is there light visible in your bedroom from the street or other sources?
- Are you often disrupted by noise whilst you sleep, or is noise generally audible from your bedroom?

If you answered 'yes' to more than one of the questions above, it is likely that your sleep quantity or quality is suboptimal. Many people do not get a sufficient amount of sleep – with time pressures from all directions, sleep is the part of life that tends to be sacrificed. Reviewing evening and morning routines may allow more time for sleeping – cutting down on television viewing, changing bath or shower schedules and re-allocating chores could all help. Refreshing sleep is particularly important to those with busy schedules, or who exercise intensively, as it allows the body to repair itself, and leads to improved energy levels.

A common occurrence is putting off going to bed during the week in order to have more time to oneself in the evening – when most of the day is swallowed up with living by externally-imposed schedules it is natural to want to carry out tasks at a leisurely pace later in the day. Regularly finding yourself surfing the internet, rearranging a bookshelf or tidying up past midnight could mean you may benefit from making time for yourself in other ways, though. A good night's sleep may enable earlier waking, more efficient working and subsequently a more relaxed evening. Rearranging a work schedule might also be useful – or if drawing out the evening is a way of extending the part of the day spent away from a dreaded workplace – a different occupation.

As well as making sure that sleep is sufficiently long in duration, it is important that the sleep is of a high quality, ideally uninterrupted and in a dark, quiet room given over to rest, that is kept at an appropriate temperature. In any given night, cycling between different sleep states occurs several times, corresponding to differing patterns of electrical activity in the brain. All of these states are required for optimal sleep, as each is associated with particular patterns of hormonal activity. When sleep is interrupted, insufficient time may be spent during specific states, and so it is possible to sleep a full 8 hours but awake feeling unrefreshed, because the sleep has been of a poorer quality and regeneration processes were not able to take place.

Certain phases of sleep bring about memory consolidation, others involve growth hormone release. In adults, growth hormone is thought to be important for preventing fat gain and increasing strength. Thus poor quality sleep can lead to difficulty with recall, and it is also associated with obesity.

The following section provides information and tips on optimising sleep, and also covers specific sleep-related disorders.

General optimization of sleep

Everyone can benefit from improving sleep quality with the following simple "sleep hygiene" points:

- Try to have a fixed time for going to bed and getting up, keeping to this at weekends and on holiday too
- Do not drink caffeine in the evening, and avoid excessive alcohol and heavy meals before bed. Do not drink any liquids immediately before bed, to avoid having to wake up to urinate
- Whilst ensuring enough physical activity is important for promoting sleep, do not exercise late in the evening, as the stimulation of the body systems will mean it is difficult to get to sleep. Sex is the only form of exercise that helps sleep
- Warm baths a few hours before bed (not immediately beforehand), lavender oil products and scented candles or oils can help with relaxation
- Keep bedrooms as clutter free as possible, and avoid using them as a workspace – remove computers, phones, work papers, etc.
- Electromagnetic radiation may also be an issue for some, so keeping the number of electrical appliances in the bedroom to a minimum, and turning them off at night,

may be advisable

- The bedroom should be well ventilated and at an appropriate temperature. Slightly cooler temperatures are generally considered to be best for healthy sleep
- Consider light levels. The body is stimulated to release melatonin, the sleep hormone, as darkness approaches, so a dark room is best for sleeping – and light is required for the waking up process. The ideal conditions would be identical to those found in nature - very dark throughout the night (no artificial lights), but gradually getting lighter towards the time when waking up approaches. Better sleep may be achieved through changing blinds or curtains or using an eye mask. Similarly, ensuring exposure to sunlight or a lamp designed to emit visible light on natural frequencies will help to establish a circadian rhythm (see November chapter)
- Reduce the impact of noise with ear plugs or double glazing if necessary
- Review the mattress and general sleeping arrangements – if disturbed by pets, children or a partner, think about how this can be changed
- Introduce a wind-down ritual. Reading a book is often better than watching television, relaxing herbal teas may also be of help
- For those who wake at night, do not toss and turn or look at the clock, and try to prevent worrying about not getting back to sleep, by going into a different room and perhaps reading for a while

Food and supplements for sleep

Whilst eating a heavy meal too close to going to bed is not recommended, eating a moderately-sized carbohydrate-containing meal earlier in the evening can help to induce feelings of relaxation, as carbohydrate intake increases brain serotonin levels.

Particular herbal teas are used traditionally to aid relaxation, such as chamomile, linden blossom and melissa, and lavender is commonly used to create feelings of relaxation. Napping during the day is sometimes necessary, but can make falling asleep at night more difficult – reduce daytime sleepiness by keeping lunches light.

There are many supplements and herbal formulations that are thought to promote sleep. Whilst good sleep hygiene will help improve the sleep of many people, extra help may occasionally be required. The following are some of the supplements often used to help promote sleep. Some preparations are easily obtained and are affordable, whereas others are more specialist and expensive.

5-HTP

As well as being useful for boosting mood (see February chapter), studies have shown that 5-HTP may help to promote restful sleep. 5-HTP increases serotonin levels, and serotonin has a relaxing, "feel good" effect. This supplement should not be taken in combination with antidepressants, prescribed sleeping pills or St John's wort.

Verdict: Consider if problems with sleep and mood are concurrent, and/or if carbohydrate cravings are a problem. Easily obtained from health food shops.

Magnesium

Supplementation with magnesium can potentially improve sleep, perhaps through stimulating the inhibitory pathways in the brain, and causing relaxation and drowsiness. Additionally, magnesium can help to relax muscles and relieve cramps, which can be a cause of disrupted sleep.

Verdict: Try if insufficient magnesium is obtained from the diet (organically grown nuts, whole grains and green vegetables are good sources), or magnesium is regularly lost through intense exercise. Choose supplements containing magnesium chelates.

Herbal remedies

There is evidence that well-known remedies such as valerian and hops can improve sleep and quality of life in subjects suffering from insomnia. A combination of herbs may be superior to single herb supplements.

Verdict: May be helpful if anxiety is also a problem. Readily available from chemists and health food shops as commercial preparations (e.g., Lanes Quiet Life).

Phosphatidylserine

This is a component of cell membranes, and so is thought to improve nerve cell conduction. It may have a role to play in helping adaptation to stress, through blunting the cortisol (stress hormone) response. It is often used by athletes to counteract the negative effects of excessive exercise, and can be helpful for promoting relaxation and sleep.

Verdict: May be of use if anxiety, stress or intense exercise contribute to the sleep problem. Not always available on the high street and relatively expensive.

L-theanine

This is an amino acid component of green tea, which inhibits the stimulatory nerve pathways in the brain, decreasing anxiety and promoting sleep. It may be useful in decreasing physiological and psychological responses to stress, thus enabling better sleep.

Verdict: Potentially helpful if anxiety is also a problem. The purified amino acid is relatively expensive, but green tea can also be used as a source

Sleep: The Chinese Medical Perspective

In Chinese medicine, *qi* (life energy) flows through specific organs at certain times of day, and so waking up at a specific time could relate to stress on a given organ.

1am – 3am – Liver. As the regulator of flow of *qi*, and the organ where Blood (which relates to more than the Western concept of the word) is stored, the Liver is central to health in Chinese medicine. Waking between these times could point to excess stress, and may co-exist with stiffness, menstrual problems, depression and IBS-type symptoms. Lifestyle modifications which reduce the amount of stress on the body may be required to restore balance.

3am – 5am – Lung. Stress on the lung may be due not only to difficulties in breathing, or a dry atmosphere, but respiration in the full sense, and thus oxidative stress. If waking at these times is a problem, ensure there is a flow of air through the room and that the temperature and humidity are optimised. Use a humidifier if necessary, consider a negative ioniser if allergies are a problem, and clear nasal passages by avoiding dairy products and performing steam inhalations. Also consider increasing consumption of vegetables and water.

5am – 7am (early waking) – Large intestine. Improper elimination may stress the large intestine, leading to waking early in the morning. Ensure an adequate intake of fibre from vegetables and legumes, as well as drinking plenty of water. Where constipation is an issue, relief can often be obtained by eating dried fruits such as prunes, or with psyllium husk drinks.

Sleep problems 1: chronic insomnia

Occasional difficulty in getting to sleep, or staying asleep is common, but a sub-section of the population has an ongoing problem with sleep, which greatly affects quality of life and ability to function.

Many cases of chronic insomnia have a mood disorder component, such as depression and anxiety. Medical problems such as asthma and gastro-intestinal reflux disease, can chronically affect sleep, as can medications. In some cases, an initial, short-lived disruption of the sleep pattern can lead to longer term insomnia – once bed becomes associated with the struggle to get to sleep, rather than with rest, more complex problems arise.

Regarding treatment of chronic insomnia, the first step is to ensure that any related medical problems are addressed appropriately. If a person can breathe easily, or has addressed their sources of anxiety, sleep may come more easily. Behavioural methods combined with good sleep hygiene can then re-set the person's daily rhythm, although this will require patience. Prescription drugs may be required, although it is best to avoid these where possible and seek gentler methods – they can be habit forming, and often there is a "hang over" or amnesiac effect.

Sleep problems 2: snoring

This common problem is caused by partial obstruction of the airways, leading to turbulent and noisy air flow. Obstruction can be from the airway tissues themselves, pressure from fat, enlarged tonsils or adenoids, or a blocked nose.

Treating underlying nose/throat conditions and ensuring the bedroom is appropriately humidified can help to minimize snoring. Losing weight and behavioural modification, such as encouraging sleep on the side, raising the head with pillows and avoiding alcohol before bed may also be helpful.

Devices to help open the airways are easy to obtain, and range from tape to keep the nasal passages open, to gumshield-like pieces of equipment which move the jaw forward. Many people find these useful.

Sleep problems 3: sleep apnoea

Sleep apnoea is a disorder where the sleeper momentarily stops breathing, on several occasions during the night. The person may snore (although snoring does not always mean sleep apnoea is present), and will most likely also suffer from daytime drowsiness and poorer mental functioning.

The most common cause of sleep apnoea is obstruction of the airway, and so increasing age and obesity are risk factors, as is smoking. Central sleep apnoea has a different cause, in that the feedback mechanisms in the central nervous system that stimulate breathing in response to rising carbon dioxide levels, do not function. A mixed picture, with elements of both obstruction and central depression, is also possible.

Diagnosis of the condition is with a sleep study. Weight loss, smoking cessation and management of other medical conditions are all first line interventions, along with behavioural techniques, such as not sleeping on the back. Positive airways pressure technology (where the airway is kept open by the application of a positively pressurized air flow) and surgery are other options, although research has now suggested that treatment with drugs such as fluoxetine can be helpful in managing the condition. Alternative approaches include the use of 5-HTP.

Sleep problems 4: restless limbs

Restless limbs syndrome is the urge to move the limbs, particularly the legs, at rest to relieve feelings of discomfort. The condition tends to run in families, and low iron stores and/or dysfunction in the dopamine (a chemical involved in nerve transmission) system may be the cause. The first step in managing this condition is treating any iron deficiency. Medically, dopamine agonists, opiates or benzodiazepines (e.g., Valium) may then be prescribed. Alternative approaches again include treatment with 5-HTP, although there is no direct evidence for the efficacy of this supplement in restless legs syndrome, Trialling a therapy such as 5-HTP once iron stores have been assessed and optimized, may be preferable to starting a hypnotic drug straight away, though.

There is anecdotal evidence that magnesium supplementation, taken orally or applied topically as an oil, can be helpful for restless limbs, as it also helpful for cramp.

Putting your mind to work

During winter, it is natural to want to shut down, physically and mentally in order to conserve energy. This is quite natural, and is mirrored in the animal and plant worlds, with some species of animal hibernating, and plants storing energy as tubers during the colder months.

The preceding chapters covered practical ways to make a new start for the body. In April, make the most of the feeling of re-awakening, and benefit from making a fresh start mentally, too.

Mental spring cleaning

Spring cleaning of your environment removes the essence of winter, and makes space for the lighter part of the year. Similarly, mental spring cleaning can be helpful in removing attitudes that detrimentally affect wellbeing, and can make it easier to maintain a healthier way of life.

Examples of attitudes which complicate wellbeing and fat loss plans:

- "If I don't achieve my goals, then I am a failure"
- "If I don't stick to my diet or exercise plan even for a day, then it has failed"
- "I need to look a certain way in order to be happy"
- "I must always control what I eat – I need to eat in a certain way"

Addressing such attitudes is not always simple, and may involve analysing their origins. A person who has succeeded in their career by being conscientious and disciplined may extend these qualities to controlling their eating or exercise habits. Whilst a certain degree of commitment in these areas is helpful and necessary, focusing too hard on perfection can be counter-productive.

Society's obsession with physical appearance can often lead to over-emphasis on achieving a particular look. Wanting to look one's best, or even wishing to change one's appearance through, for example, losing weight can be healthy, as achieving these goals usually requires an all-round improved lifestyle – but strongly associating happiness with achieving a particular appearance can cause many problems. Use the workbook space at the end of this chapter to start exploring which attitudes need to be modified or swept away entirely, in order to make progress.

New ideas and new projects

As the days lengthen, you may feel as though you have more time, and April is a great month to begin new projects. Make a list of things you would like to try – this might include learning a new language, taking up a hobby, overhauling your home or garden, trying a sport or visiting a particular country. Then work out which of these would be possible this year. Be adventurous!

Buy, or make, a book to jot down ideas as they arise, now that nature has awoken, you might find you feel more inspired in many areas of your life. This could be the year where you make some great changes.

Chapter summary

- Build on new starts made in March this month, and have a healthier Easter - a little planning and some alternatives to chocolate can make a big difference
- Ensure your body has opportunities for renewal through healthy sleep every night. Make your bedroom dark and quiet, and start a wind-down ritual. Certain supplements can help if relaxing in the evening is a problem

- Explore new opportunities and address unhelpful beliefs to make the most of the season of growth

Workbook section

My plans for Easter:

How this Easter will be healthier than in previous years:

Steps I will take to improve sleep:

New things I will introduce into my life this month:

Ideas for new projects:

Make a note of any unhelpful beliefs around fat loss and healthy living, where these came from and how they could be addressed. For example:

Belief: Healthy eating is boring

Where did this come from? Being on restrictive diets

Action: Make an effort to cook interesting healthy meals and try out new ingredients

Summer

Development
Beauty
Enjoyment

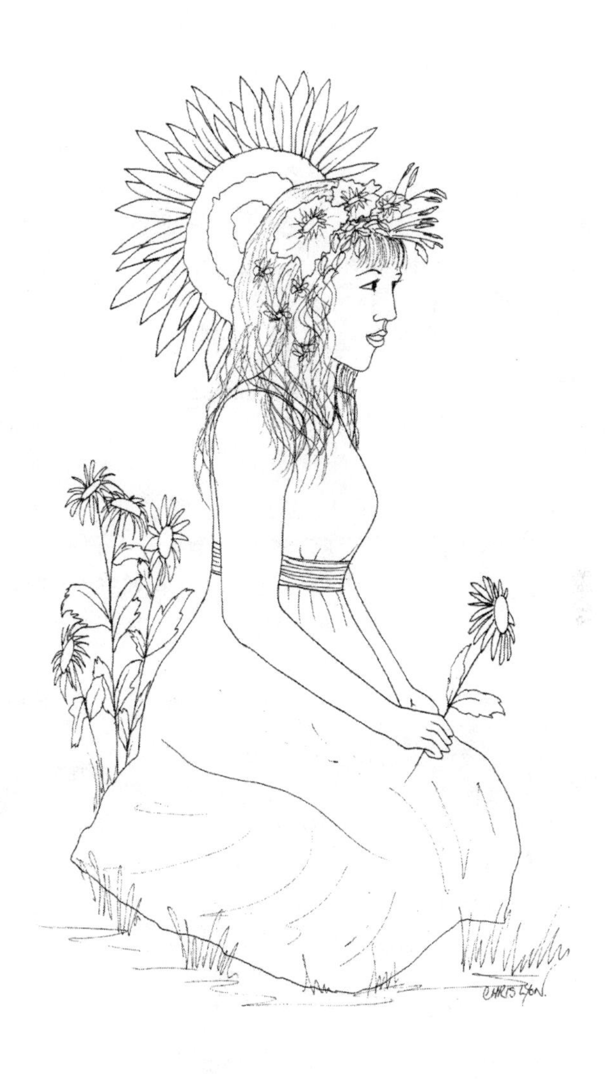

May

Love, joy, beauty

The start of May was celebrated as the start of summer in many European countries, with the Celtic festival of Beltane being well documented in Ireland and Scotland. This is a festival of fire, which may have evolved from smoke-treatment of livestock, to reduce the risk of disease. May rituals involving fire are also found in the Czech Republic, where effigies of witches are burned to drive out winter, and in Germany (Walpurgis night), again associated with witches.

In England, the May celebrations were key social occasions, involving dances round the maypole, feasting, and the displaying and selling of May flower garlands. Maypoles were permanent and important features of English villages for several centuries although their popularity waned with increasing urbanisation. Claims that maypole dancing involves phallic symbolism are thought to be unfounded.

Flowers and the month of May have always been connected - from the Roman Floralia festival, in honour of the goddess Flora, who protected flowers and blossoms, to the flower garland displays, which were a part of May celebrations in England until the 20th century.

The origin of the month's name in English could be from the Roman goddess Maia, or from maiores, meaning older men (with June being dedicated to Juno or juniores, young men). In the Anglo-Saxon calendar, the month corresponding to May was Thrimilci, "three milkings", perhaps because the production of large amounts of dairy products could take place during this period. The non-Latin name of the month translates as flower month (Czech), grass month (Ukrainian, Belarusian), and budding month (Croatian).

A Bank Holiday in the UK, 1 May is a workers' holiday in

many countries, and also celebrated as International Workers' Day, or Labour Day. The second bank holiday in the UK is around the date (29 May) that Restoration Day, or Royal Oak Day was marked in the past. This date was set aside as a national holiday to celebrate the restoration of the monarchy, the oak being significant as King Charles II took refuge inside an oak tree to escape his pursuers. Even after political changes caused the removal of the event from the list of public holidays, it was marked by individuals, particularly children, and communities by the wearing of foliage.

The ecclesiastical festivals of Ascension Day, Rogationtide and Pentecost often fall in May. The Rogationtide custom of blessing the crops echoes the Roman festival of Ambarvalia, where sacrifices were made to protect crops.

May is a month to celebrate and enjoy the beauty of nature, and to hope for its continued blessings. Events in the past such as the May games and the crowning of the May Kings and Queens encouraged communities to come together, and national holidays have been aspects of the cultural calendar for centuries. Today, the two bank holidays in the UK during this month encourage us to relax. Living a healthier lifestyle feels easier now– comfort food is less of a requirement, and being active is a pleasure, rather than a chore.

May day celebrations were considered opportunities for young couples to meet, and warnings that maidens who went out to celebrate the coming of May often ended up pregnant were commonplace. In the Czech Republic, May 1 is still celebrated as a day for lovers.

Hayfever

Unfortunately, the joy of spring and summer can be overshadowed by hayfever. Relief can be provided by antihistamines and decongestant sprays, with more severe cases requiring corticosteroids. There are a number of natural remedies which can help reduce hayfever symptoms, and the need for medication.

Local honey

There are no studies on whether regularly using honey can prevent hayfever, but anecdotal evidence abounds. The proposed mechanism is that honey contains small amounts of the pollen that can cause hay fever, and so eating it desensitises the immune system, meaning there is less reaction to airborne pollen. Local honey is the best option as it should contain the pollen that is also causing symptoms (regional is local enough in the UK).

Verdict: Natural and generally safe. Best to start before the hayfever season. May not be the best option for those looking to lose fat.

Marshmallow root

Studies have shown that this herb, used as a folk remedy for hayfever, can protect the mucosa and also suppress cough, although there are no studies specifically showing reductions of hayfever symptoms directly.

Verdict: Little direct evidence, but easy to obtain.

Removing the pollen, or preventing it from reaching the lining of the nose

Creating a barrier against the pollen with a powder or gel can be effective in reducing the amount of pollen reaching the lining of the nose. There are no studies on salt water sprays, but common sense would indicate that removing pollen from the nose by washing would be helpful.

Verdict: Avoiding contact between the pollen and the mucosa makes sense for hay fever sufferers. This starts with changing clothes after spending time outdoors and showering before bed. Pollen barriers may help, as may salt water nasal sprays.

Perilla

Extracts of this herb have been shown to reduce symptoms in a small group of hayfever sufferers. Its active ingredient, rosmarinic acid, was also shown to be effective when purified and used alone.

Verdict: A promising-sounding option, but further research may be needed. Also, not easy to obtain on the high street.

Probiotics

As well as having other health benefits, certain probiotics have been shown to reduce hayfever symptoms in a number of studies. It is important to use a good quality probiotic containing *L.acidophilus* and *B.lactis* (the product should state the activity level and give an expiry date) – inferior products and sugary "probiotic" drinks are less likely to be effective. Alternatively you may wish to try a natural source of friendly bacteria, such as kefir, a fermented milk drink, although dosage and activity level is less assured with these.

Verdict: Definitely worth a try – there is evidence to support use and probiotics have many other benefits.

Quercetin

There are a small number of studies showing the effectiveness of modified quercetin and of a formula containing (amongst other components) quercetin for reducing hayfever symptoms. Quercetin is related chemically to cromolyn, a compound used medically to treat allergies and asthma.

Verdict: Again, promising, but more studies are needed. Anecdotal evidence seems to be strong, and the product is easily obtained. Quercetin is present in many foods, including apples, onions and tea and can be bought as a supplement.

Nasal phototherapy

This method has been shown to reduce hay fever symptoms, and the mechanism of action may involve regulation of immune system stimulation by the UV light. The dose of light used is unlikely to cause long-term DNA damage, but the longer term effects of the therapy are yet to be studied.

Verdict: Increasingly available, and some proven efficacy. May be an option for those with more severe symptoms, or when other methods have not helped.

Acupuncture

Opinions are divided as to the efficacy of acupuncture for hay fever, and results are awaited from large trials, which may help clarify the situation.

Verdict: Often easy to obtain, and may be worthwhile trying if symptoms are severe or not easily controlled, as it tends to be a cost effective with few side effects.

Time for love and sex

The associations between May and romantic love and sex are not surprising. Flowers, linked with the time of year, are in fact part of a plant's reproductive system, and the exuberance of nature and the improved weather encourages us to connect with others.

Specifically, thoughts may turn to sexual expression. From a physical perspective, maintaining a healthy weight/body fat percentage, taking regular exercise and optimising sleep will all contribute to an improved sex life. Supplements generally believed to help enhance sexual performance/experience are discussed below. Overall, whilst physiology does undoubtedly have a part to play, psychological and interpersonal factors are likely to be more important.

Zinc

Supplementing with zinc may be generally useful, as deficiency is common, and zinc deficiency can cause a variety of problems including sexual dysfunction in men. Zinc supplementation also improves sperm quality in men with sub-optimal sperm. However, using zinc supplementation to boost testosterone levels, sexual desire or sexual performance in men or women is not supported by evidence, and how zinc affects the male reproductive system is not known.

Verdict: Correcting deficiency is important, and supplementation may improve fertility in males, but unlikely to have a direct effect on sexual desire or performance.

Horny goat weed (epimedium)

This herb is used as a Chinese therapy for erectile dysfunction, although there is little clinical research into its effects in humans. Its active component is icariin, which has been shown, when chemically modified, to have a similar mechanism of action to Viagra.

Verdict: The evidence is not strong, but there is a long history of usage. May be helpful if erectile dysfunction specifically is the main problem, and obtaining a formulation after consultation with a practitioner of Chinese medicine may lead to better results than using a shop-bought variety.

Gingko biloba

Extracts of this plant have been shown to improve blood flow, and there is evidence for its usefulness in dementia. Seeing as blood flow to the vagina and clitoris is important for sexual arousal in women, it was trialled as a therapy for women with sexual arousal disorder. There was little support for the use of the herb for this indication – although it is possible that the conduction of the study itself may have had an inhibitory effect on sexual arousal.

Verdict: A herb with proven benefits, but perhaps not in the field of sexual dysfunction.

Tribulus terrestris
This herb, used in Eastern medicine, is now widely promoted in fitness circles as being capable of increasing strength and lean mass, through its effects on testosterone, although there is little scientific evidence for this.

Verdict: Little evidence to support its ability to act as an aphrodisiac or improve sexual function in humans.

Maca
Native to Peru, this root is purported to optimise sex hormone balance in men and women, improving sexual performance, fertility, memory and mood. Preparations are available for perimenopausal women, and it is also marketed as an energy booster. There is little scientific research on maca, although preliminary research showed it increased sexual desire and sporting performance in male cyclists.

Verdict: May be a promising supplement, but not enough evidence to support its use. There may also be significant variation in preparations.

Contraception - working with your hormones

Discussion of sex may lead to consideration of contraception. For women, the use of hormonal contraception merits particular focus. Whilst the pill is convenient and reliable, with a number of added benefits depending on the formulation, prolonged use should perhaps be questioned. The decision to change the method of contraception should not be taken lightly, and should be discussed within the couple as well as with healthcare providers. Some of the risks and benefits of the pill, as well as issues with ceasing hormonal contraception are summarised below.

Benefits of hormonal contraceptive pills:

- Reliable, easy to use contraceptive

- Reduced risk of ovarian cancer (combined pill)
- Reduced risk of endometrial cancer
- Reduced PMS
- Certain formulations can be used to treat acne
- Possible to "control" periods
- Reliable, convenient form of contraception
- Reduction in symptoms of endometriosis and polycystic ovary syndrome

Risks/negatives of hormonal contraceptive pills:

- Taking a pill is easy to forget
- Slightly increased risk of breast cancer (combined pill), disappears 5-10 years after stopping use
- Increased risk of cervical cancer with long term use
- Increased risk of benign liver tumours and liver cancer in current users
- Increased risk of venous thrombosis (combined pill, current users)
- Potential to increase blood pressure
- Potential to cause side effects including skin problems, hair loss, irregular periods, changes in mood and libido, headaches and nausea
- Research does not support the commonly-held belief that pill usage leads to fat gain – although anecdotally, this has been the experience of many women
- Use can lead to depletion of nutrients such as b vitamins, selenium and zinc and increased oxidative stress
- After long-term use, it may take some time for fertility and normal menstrual pattern to be restored
- Environmental impact – women using the pill produce hormone-rich urine. The excreted hormones may affect aquatic life, and may also contribute to the pollution of drinking water with oestrogens

Issues with ceasing to use hormonal contraceptive pills

- Increased risk of pregnancy – necessary to find a new method of contraception
- Possibility of hair loss, worsening skin conditions and worsening PMS
- Menstrual cycle can take months to regulate after stopping use of the pill

Natural methods of contraception may be an option for those in long-term relationships. If such a method is chosen, it is important to understand that avoiding sex for the few days around ovulation (e.g., the rhythm method) is not sufficient if pregnancy is to be prevented. Sperm can survive in the female genital tract for several days, and the egg cell, once released, also survives for several days. Investing in a hormone monitor, such as Persona, will help to identify days when pregnancy could potentially occur. Basal temperature measurements and assessment of cervical mucus are other methods that could be used to gauge the balance of hormones on a particular day, although temperature measurements may be affected by the amount of time spent sleeping, whether the woman engaged in exercise, alcohol intake and other factors, and cervical mucus assessment does not appeal to everyone.

The withdrawal method is not generally considered to be effective, as the common belief is that pre-ejaculatory fluid contains sperm. However, few studies have been carried out into this area, and some researchers suggest that pre-ejaculatory fluid does not contain sperm. When performed correctly, the withdrawal method may be a contraceptive option for some couples, particularly when combined with other forms of monitoring – although it is perhaps not to be recommended where avoiding pregnancy is of utmost importance.

No method of contraception is 100% reliable, and there is a perception that natural methods are more fallible, perhaps because there is a greater margin for human error. Many couples find natural methods highly effective, and prefer a form of family planning that does not impact on the body or on the environment. Natural methods are best suited to those in long-term supportive relationships, where communication around sex and around the risk of pregnancy is not an issue.

Neither natural nor hormonal methods of contraception provide any protection against sexually transmitted diseases such as chlamydia, gonorrhea, HIV and syphilis.

Feeling great this season

It is now that many people want to lose weight, look their best and sparkle. After the invigorating, but unpredictable, start to spring, May is often the month when the first warm days are experienced, meaning we want to be outdoors and socialise.

Starting diet and lifestyle changes earlier in the year will allow results to be seen by summer, but if a programme never got off the ground, make the most of new-found enthusiasm and start now. Review earlier chapters – you might wish to start with some of the "detox" ideas in the March chapter.

Other factors to consider when preparing for summer are skin and hair. Many of us have significant personal esteem invested into the appearance of these parts of the body – perhaps not surprising, since they are often considered barometers of health. A person with hormones in balance, with an optimal intake of nutrients and water, should have healthy, shiny hair and clear, radiant skin. Appearances can be transformed by a new hair style, and the uncertainty of adolescence can re-emerge due to a skin breakout. The following tips, in addition to a generally healthy lifestyle will help to support the condition of hair and skin.

Skin

Most adolescents experience some form of acne, and adult acne is increasingly common. Adult skin breakouts are often related to hormonal imbalances – changes in the skin around menstruation are familiar to a significant proportion of women – and more severe problems can occur due to Polycystic Ovarian Syndrome (PCOS) (involving excess androgens), or may have no apparent cause. Stress can also cause breakouts, as can certain skin care products.

If you have recently begun to develop severe acne, and this is distressing, see your doctor, who may suggest further tests, including those for PCOS. The typical symptoms of PCOS include being overweight (and finding it very difficult to lose weight), acne, excess hair on the face and body, and insulin resistance, although not all of these characteristics need to be present. Many women with PCOS are slim. Diagnosis may involve ultrasound, which in PCOS can show multiple cysts on the ovaries (corresponding to abnormal ovulation), androgen assessment and glucose tolerance testing.

Whether acne is severe, moderate or mild, improving diet and lifestyle can often be helpful. The link between diet and skin has been a point of debate, but there is now considerable evidence for the role of dairy products and high GI foods (sweets and refined carbohydrates) in acne and the formation of breakouts – avoiding these completely may lead to significant improvements. Even PCOS may be ameliorated by a low GI or low carbohydrate diet.

There are a number of supplements that may help to improve skin condition. Probiotics have been shown to inhibit growth of the bacterium responsible for acne in a laboratory setting, and as ensuring an optimal balance of gut flora helps with many aspects of wellbeing, starting a probiotic may be generally worthwhile. Omega-3 fatty acids have a role to play in skin health, and are suggested as adjunct treatments for a wide range of skin disorders, from acne to psoriasis and atopic eczema. Maintaining adequate vitamin D levels may be helpful for treating acne and proliferative skin disorders, and zinc has long been suggested as key for managing acne.

Whilst the causes of acne usually come from within the body, reviewing skin care products may help to at least reduce redness and irritation. Throw away old make-up and clean out your makeup bag or box and if you regularly use foundation or powder, perhaps trial a few weeks without it.

You might also wish to try the natural, oil absorbing products specifically for acne-prone skin. Whilst many "miracle" skin care products are no more effective than the simplest creams and lotions, certain brands have an excellent reputation, and may be helpful. Consider consulting with a skincare professional or dermatologist to ensure you choose the right products – many people make the mistake of choosing overly harsh products, which further irritate the skin. You may benefit from a very gentle, all-natural product that reduces stress on the skin. Finally, there are over-the-counter preparations that can be helpful for acne, such as Freederm and Quinoderm.

Preventing skin ageing

Whilst sun exposure is the most natural way to maintain healthy vitamin D levels, and the connection between sun exposure and malignant melanoma may not be as simple as we are led to believe, excessive sun exposure does lead to skin ageing (see July chapter).

There are concerns over the ingredients of some sun protection creams and lotions, and if you wish to protect your skin as much as possible but prefer not to use these on a regular basis, avoiding the sun may be the best option – cover up, and use a broad brimmed hat or parasol to reduce exposure of the face. Avoiding the sun in this way may mean vitamin D supplementation is required.

Additionally, eat as naturally as possible, and be sure to

include a wide range of vegetables every day, to provide the phytochemicals required to reduce stress on the body. Make an effort to drink plenty of water, perhaps having certain times of the day where a certain amount is drunk, keep alcohol intake to a minimum, and if you smoke, cut down or better still, quit. Where possible, avoid passive smoking and other sources of pollution.

Natural skin products may be the best option for longer-term skin health; there are concerns over whether synthetic varieties can actually do more damage than they claim to prevent.

Hair

Loss of hair is unpleasant for both men and women – for men, though, it is an accepted part of growing older. In women, it can signal a nutrient imbalance or a hormonal problem, and can be extremely distressing.

Hair loss in women usually takes a different pattern to male hair loss, being more generalised. Often, it is caused by telogen effluvium – which refers to the phase of hair growth (telogen) and to mass shedding of hair (effluvium). Changes in the balance of female hormones, iron deficiency and hypothyroidism can all lead to telogen effluvium. Of these, iron deficiency and hypothyroidism can be easily diagnosed and treated in a straightforward way, although re-growth of hair will take some months. If you are suffering from hair loss, see your doctor. Your blood tests should include ferritin, as well as haemoglobin. If iron levels are low, you may be prescribed iron supplements – there are also iron-based supplements for female hair loss available in over the counter preparations, too.

Female hair loss is common after giving birth, due to the sudden decline in hormone levels. A similar situation may be observed with stopping the contraceptive pill. The shedding of the hair actually signifies that a new hair is ready to grow, and eventually, if the hormones are allowed to re-set, the hair will thicken. Supporting the body with good nutrition, adequate rest and exercise will be helpful here, as well as dealing with any psychological outcomes of the hair loss. A well-known supplement, purported to help with hair loss is the marine-based Nourkrin; several months are required for effects to be seen.

Another cause of hair loss is extreme dieting. If you wish to lose weight (fat), going about this in a controlled manner will not only prevent such side effects, but is more likely to lead to longer-term maintenance of your target weight (body fat percentage). Losing weight should be part of a healthier lifestyle – not a quick fix.

Female menstrual problems

Many women accept Premenstrual Syndrome (PMS) as a fact of life, and whilst some cramping, changes in mood, etc. are perhaps to be expected due to the changes in hormone levels, major disruptions should not be accepted as "normal". Whilst PMS can be tackled year-round, addressing it when we want to rid ourselves of limiting influences and enjoy life to the full, seems appropriate.

On the first day of a period, levels of all hormones are low. Over the first part of the cycle, until ovulation (the release of an egg cell from an ovary), which is roughly half-way through, levels of oestrogen begin to increase, as egg follicles develop in the ovary. This is in response to Follicle Stimulating Hormone (FSH), a signal from the brain. Oestrogen, produced mostly by the ovaries, has a number of actions, including building up the lining of the womb, and increasing energy levels and optimism.

When levels of oestrogen are sufficiently high, Luteinising Hormone (LH) is secreted from the brain's pituitary gland, causing the release of an egg from a follicle. Oestrogen levels start to decline, and the egg is then propelled to the womb, via the Fallopian tube, where if sperm is present, it is fertilised –

otherwise it dies.

The left-over follicle (which could be thought of as a tiny, soft egg shell) secretes the hormone progesterone, which has further preparatory effects on the lining of the womb, having a variety of other effects throughout the body. After about a week, the follicle begins to degrade, and progesterone levels decrease (unless fertilisation of an egg has taken place), which may be part of the cause of the irritability and water retention symptoms of PMS. The lining of the womb is no longer "supported" by hormones, and falls away as a menstrual period.

A "negative feedback" system acts here, as well as elsewhere – a stimulatory hormone from a master gland (such as the pituitary in the brain) acts on a gland elsewhere in the body to release the effector hormone - in the case of the menstrual cycle, oestrogen. Rising levels of the effector hormone then provide the signal to cease production of the stimulatory hormone – which helps to ensure levels of all hormones remain in the optimal range. During menstruation, the levels of the effector hormones such as oestrogen are low, causing release of the stimulatory hormones from the brain. This is a simplified picture, and feedback loops can be more complex, with the "stimulatory" hormones also having direct effects on body tissues.

It is clear from even this short description that the menstrual cycle involves a number of carefully-orchestrated changes. In addition to the hormonal changes, alterations in neurotransmitter balance and other chemical messengers also occur, which combined with lifestyle factors, can contribute to PMS.

Due to the inter-related nature of hormones, making adjustments to diet and supplementation may help to reduce the impact of hormonal changes on the body. Many women find that reducing intake of caffeine, alcohol and refined carbohydrate and including more natural foods may help reduce symptoms, as may avoiding exogenous sources of oestrogens such as plastics and dairy products. An optimal intake of water and fibre will support the elimination of hormones from the body, and you may wish to consider supporting good nutrition with supplements of vitamins and minerals, if you suffer from PMS.

The impact of soy isoflavones on female hormonal balance is unclear, although sufficient controversy exists to warrant avoiding large intakes – soy may also have an impact on the thyroid. Soy is cited as a reason for lower breast cancer incidence in Far Eastern countries, although the situation is not so straight forward. The Western use of soy products also differs greatly from the traditional use – soy milk, soy "meat" and suchlike are Western inventions, and soy is rarely used in the Far East as a major protein source, more as an accompaniment to a meal, and often in fermented form.

Agnus Castus (also known as Vitex Agnus Castus, Vitex and Chasteberry) has been used by women for centuries to ease menstrual symptoms, and whilst it has not been extensively researched in a laboratory setting, there are a number of studies supporting its efficacy, including a randomised, placebo controlled, prospective trial, published in the the prestigious British Medical Journal in 2001.

Trials for magnesium supplementation for PMS have been promising (although the type of magnesium supplement used is important – magnesium oxide, the most commonly available form, was not shown to be effective), and whilst there is little evidence for the use of evening primrose in PMS generally, it has been shown in a pilot study to reduce breast pain, which is often part of PMS. Vitamin E also had a similar effect. Overall, the best-supported herbal supplement for PMS is Agnus Castus, and a trial of this herb may be warranted if you want to decrease your PMS symptoms.

Chapter summary

- Enjoy the beauty of May without hayfever - examine natural options for prevention and relief, such as marshmallow root and perilla

- Consider how your sex life and your contraceptive options can be optimised
- Try out food and supplements to support the health of your skin and hair, and to fight PMS, so you are looking and feeling your best. Agnus castus can help with pre-menstrual symptoms and also with skin, as many adult skin problems are hormone related

Workbook section

Associations this time of year has for me:

Ideas for preventing or relieving hayfever:

Thoughts on sex and/or contraception:

How I will support the health of my skin and hair:

PMS action plan:

June

The halfway point

The midpoint of the year, and the month in which the middle of summer is considered to fall, is full of warmth and light, popular today for gatherings of many kinds – garden parties, barbecues, weddings. The name of the month in English is thought to derive from the goddess Juno, or to be related to young men (juniores). In other languages, the name of the month is červen, (Czech, Ukrainian, Belarusian, Polish meaning red – referring to the ripening of fruits) or lipanj (Croatian, month of the linden tree).

The summer solstice in the northern hemisphere takes place on 21 June. This represents the northern hemisphere being closest to the sun, and where there is little change in the position of the sun as seen from Earth. This is the lightest part of the year – days are at their longest.

The church feast of Corpus Christi takes place this month, and this was an important occasion for drama productions for several centuries. Still more significant are the fire celebrations at midsummer. These took place on 24 June, which is both midsummer day and St John's day, as well as on 28 June, the eve of the feast of saints Peter and Paul. St John's day is celebrated with fires all across Europe. The origin of the ceremony is believed to be pre-Christian, and related to protection, with the earliest record of Midsummer fire celebration dating from the 4th century.

English midsummer celebrations included either burning wheels or festive fires, as well as processions, singing, dancing and feasting – food and drink would be provided by wealthier members of the community. In some cases, elaborate spectacles would be arranged. Once the fire had burned down, young men would leap over the flames in a contest of bravery. Young girls and then married women would later do the same, for luck, and finally cattle would be walked through the remains of the fire.

In Russia, Ukraine, Belarus and Poland, the St John's Eve feast brings in the element of water as well as fire, perhaps as it honours St John the Baptist (Ivan Kupala). Unmarried women make garlands of flowers, and float them in a river – the behaviour of the garlands can be used to predict relationships. A young man can attract a girl's attention by capturing her wreath. St John's Eve is associated with magic – the folk belief that the fern flower blooms on this evening is described in Nikolai Gogol's story, "St John's Eve" – picking the flower confers supernatural powers.

In England, shearing sheep and harvesting hay and rushes would have all taken place in June. In the north west of the country, a ritual element was attached to the rush harvest. Whilst the hottest months are typically yet to come, the conditions of maximum light are achieved during June. After this, perhaps imperceptibly to begin with, the light begins to wane, and flowers and leaves begin to give way to fruits. Growth and new life is replaced by maturation and ripening, and ultimately by decay and storage. This is reflected in Robert Graves' poetic description of the Holly King and the Oak King, two aspects of a male seasonal deity who engaged in battles at midsummer and midwinter. The Holly King, who rules the darker part of the year, prevails at midsummer, and the Oak King prevails at midwinter; thus the origin of winter is already perceived in summer, and deepest winter is when nature is preparing for summer. This concept would have had a practical application for agrarian societies – preparation of the ground in winter was key for ensuring a harvest, and care must be taken to nurture and protect crops in summer to provide food throughout the colder months.

By now, new lifestyle habits should be established, and it should be possible to "harvest" some of the first rewards of improved lifestyle and self-awareness from earlier in the year.

During June, review these habits and consider whether increasing intensity and focus is now required.

Moving to the next level

The middle of the season and the middle of the year represented a transition for farming communities – sowing is complete, growth is taking place, and the next part of the cycle, which includes maintaining and then harvesting crops was about to begin. Review your motivations, practices and progress now.

Why changes may be needed

It is necessary to regularly review fat loss plans, since the body adapts to styles of eating and exercise to conserve energy. There is no evolutionary advantage to deliberately losing fat – the ability to store fat efficiently would have been useful for early humans, who faced regular periods of low food availability. Contrast this, and the greater levels of activity of previous generations, with the abundance of readily-available energy dense-foods in developed countries and the sedentary lifestyles led by many people, and it is possible to draw the conclusion that halting the obesity epidemic in the West will require a re-alignment of the environment and human genetic programming.

For general wellbeing, as the body heals, a different plan may be required – in the early stages of correcting a functional imbalance, it may be necessary to supplement the diet with specific micronutrients. Once balance has been restored and healthy eating habits established, the number of supplements required can decrease. Conversely, increasing exercise intensity and the progression to regular sports training may require the introduction of new supplements to support the body in dealing with the demands of more intense training.

The following list gives some ideas as to how plans may be adapted. Use the space at the end of the chapter to record your thoughts.

- Moving from activity and regular exercise to progressive training and perhaps taking advice from a fitness professional, or booking a block of sessions to get started (See References chapter for advice on choosing a gym and a Personal trainer)
- Increasing the number of training sessions per week
- Committing to regular sports skill training sessions, if you have started to take an interest in sport
- Consulting a nutrition/wellbeing professional about your diet or any specific concerns
- Adapting your nutrition plan as you achieve results and re-align your goals
- Making appointments with your GP or other healthcare advisor to discuss specific medical problems
- Committing to eat more organically and locally, using Farmers' Markets on a regular basis, etc.(See August chapter)
- Reviewing your supplementation plan. Could you benefit from adding a new supplement, or conversely, do you feel you are taking too many supplements?

Adapting your nutrition plan

Restriction and re-introduction

Grains only became part of the diet with the advent of agriculture, and now – usually in processed form, they make up the majority of the Western diet (see September chapter). Cutting back on refined carbohydrates helps with fat loss and wellbeing, and greater carbohydrate restriction, including removal of even whole grains and legumes from the menu, or committing to eating only the foods that would have been available to hunter-gatherers (e.g., the Paleo diet, based on protein, vegetables, fruit and nuts, with no dairy or grains) can also be helpful for fat loss, although this may not need to be continued in the longer term.

Carbohydrate restriction or Paleo eating in the early stages of a fat loss plan has benefits beyond the metabolic – it can act as a mental "detox". cutting out grains and dairy will automatically mean removing refined and fast foods. To begin with, this will present practical difficulties, as it becomes clear that the majority of readily available foods are not part of the eating plan. Eventually, new strategies will be developed – carrying nuts or apples for snacks, preparing meals in advance, creating "portable" meals. Shops and restaurants providing appropriate foods will be noted.

Additionally, removing foods such as wheat or dairy from the diet may reveal an underlying intolerance – avoiding the culprits then becomes logical, and does not feel like deprivation. Many foods can cause intolerances, some of the other common culprits include fish, nuts, eggs and legumes. Whilst unnecessarily cutting out food groups for long periods is not advisable, and true food allergy is relatively rare, sensitisation to food components is common. This can occur when a particular food is eaten too frequently, or may be due to an individual's metabolic constitution. Intolerances can be subtle, and variable. For example, it may be possible to eat a certain amount of nuts, contained in a meal, but eating a handful alone could lead to feelings of discomfort.

Whilst it is not healthy to have a continual mental focus on food, or to eat in an overly controlled way, having a nutrition plan for several months will help not only with fat loss, but if designed correctly, will lead to the formation of new habits. Once these habits are formed, the healthier style of eating will be automatic.

Additionally, after initial restriction of food types, whether for fat loss or wellbeing purposes, foods can gradually be re-introduced, and may even be required. One drawback of a low carbohydrate diet is that it can lead to lethargy in some, but not all, active individuals. Introducing unprocessed carbohydrates back into the diet can assist with an intense training regime. Re-introduction may not be successful though, – it may become clear that including wheat in the diet has more disadvantages than advantages, for example.

Timing

Timing of meals and particular macronutrients can be important, due to the effects of the components of food on particular hormones. Whilst too much consideration of food as a collection of nutrients is unhelpful, it is worthwhile keeping in mind some key ideas.

Carbohydrate-rich meals cause a large insulin response (especially refined or simple carbohydrates) and an increase in brain serotonin, which can produce both feelings of happiness and relaxation/lethargy. Eating a carbohydrate-rich breakfast may thus not be the best option for alertness and mental performance throughout the morning.

For those that exercise, carbohydrate consumption following exercise, along with protein, will help to provide muscles with the raw materials they need to bring about repair and growth. Where muscle growth in particular is the aim, post-workout carbohydrate will harness the anabolic potential of insulin (the hormone is responsible for storage of nutrients, but also can stimulate muscle growth).

Overall, avoid carbohydrate-rich breakfasts, and have a minimal or moderate carbohydrate intake at lunch, depending on your needs. The main carbohydrate intake should be in the evening. For those that exercise in the morning, a solution is to include a small amount of carbohydrate post-workout – for example, a protein shake with added oats. You may need to experiment with the amount of carbohydrate – too much may cause drowsiness, and too little may lead to lower energy levels for some people.

Focusing on protein and fat at breakfast will provide amino acids and fatty acids for neurotransmitter synthesis, and will also provide satiety and energy for the morning. Rich meals later in the evening should be avoided, as these can disrupt sleep.

Ideas for planning nutrient intake for an active person:

Breakfast: Protein and fat. E.g., scrambled eggs and smoked salmon

Mid morning snack: half a handful of nuts

Lunch: Protein, vegetables and small portion of carbohydrate, e.g., a lean steak with steamed vegetables and a small serving of brown rice

Afternoon snack: an apple

Evening meal: Complex carbohydrate, vegetables, small serving of protein, e.g. small chicken breast, salad and new potatoes

Hormones and lifestyle

Hormones must be kept in balance, too little or too much of a particular major hormone is usually problematic.

Insulin is released in response to eating, with a more dramatic response to carbohydrates than other types of nutrient. Without it, nutrients cannot enter cells to be used or stored, and in the case of completely deficiency without replacement, early death usually results (as in the case of type 1 diabetics before the discovery of insulin - people with this disease require injections of insulin). Insulin is the hormone of storage and building – optimising it is important for those looking to increase muscle size. However, it is also a significant fat storage hormone – once the needs for energy have been satisfied and extra glucose stored as glycogen in the muscles and liver, any excess is stored as fat.

If insulin is stimulated excessively over the course of decades, most likely due to a diet rich in refined carbohydrates, receptors on the majority of body cells lose their sensitivity to it.

Fat cells remain sensitive to the hormone, and continue to grow and multiply, though. Insulin levels increase to counteract the decreased sensitivity on non-fat cells, and so the body gets caught in fat storage mode. The constellation of obesity, poor response to insulin, blood fat abnormalities and high blood pressure is known as the metabolic syndrome, and it increases cardiovascular risk significantly. High levels of insulin correlate with excessive general inflammation, and may also confer an increased risk of cancers and dementia. Overall, then, too little or too much insulin is dangerous.

A similar picture is seen with all hormones. A person's ability to function is affected significantly by either abnormally high or abnormally low levels of thyroid hormone. The "female" hormones oestrogen and progesterone are important for both men and women – deficiency affects fertility in both sexes, whereas excess leads to fat deposition, and an increased risk for certain cancers. Similarly, testosterone is required by both sexes, but excess in either sex leads to aggression, acne and excessive body and facial hair growth. Low levels of cortisol, the stress hormone, are part of adrenal fatigue and lead to lethargy, low morning energy, low blood pressure and inability to deal with stress, amongst other symptoms. Elevated levels of cortisol can cause abdominal obesity, increased cardiovascular risk and depression.

There is another layer of complexity: hormones can affect each other. High levels of cortisol can affect thyroid hormone function and can bring about insulin resistance.

Hormonal balance can be manipulated by food, supplements and other lifestyle aspects such as sleep and exercise. Rather than turning to expensive supplements or treatments, or difficult regimes, achieving and maintaining balance is best done by first addressing the basics, as follows:

- Optimal sleep (see April Chapter)

- Sufficient intake of good quality, clean water
- Appropriate amounts of natural foods, with an eating schedule to suit the individual and their goals
- Regular, balanced physical activity
- Stress management techniques
- Targeted supplementation

Sticking to a plan in summer

With the warmer weather come a variety of distractions from routine with frequent gatherings, centred around food and drink. Where these occur regularly, it may be necessary to consider the impact they may have on overall lifestyle and approach. Keep in mind the following:

- Set a weekly limit for alcohol and do not exceed it, no matter how many parties are expected
- Eat before attending drinks parties
- When drinking alcohol, have plenty of water too
- If you have a particularly busy social period, put exercise in the diary, as an appointment. Otherwise several weeks may go by with little physical activity. If exercising at a gym is less appealing now, consider how aspects of your training programme can be moved outdoors. Some parks have areas with fitness equipment
- Suggest making meetings with friends more active – for example having a walk before eating lunch together
- Weddings can be particularly difficult in terms of food. Many wedding services in England are held around lunch time, meaning that there is often a large gap between breakfast and the next meal. Alcohol is abundant and typical wedding foods are far from healthy. Have a filling breakfast, and take a small snack such as nuts or an apple with you, to eat between the end of the ceremony and the wedding meal. This will help to keep blood sugar levels

balanced, and will reduce the risk of over-indulging on canapés or heavily-iced wedding cake

Aches, pains and injuries

Long days and better weather can inspire increased activity, more demanding workouts and experiments with new sports. Make the most of the energy of the time of year and be as active as possible – but look out for injuries, aches and pains.

Injuries

If you have sustained a sports-related injury, there are steps that can be taken immediately to minimise discomfort and damage, including:

- Rest – avoid using the affected limb as much as possible, do not continue to exercise
- Ice
- Compression
- Elevation

The next step in treating the injury is to seek expert advice, from your GP, or Accident and Emergency department, depending on severity, and/or a physiotherapist or sports massage therapist. Injuries are usually given a few days to rest before being treated.

Unfortunately, a sports injury will impact your exercise programme, and depending on the injury, may require lengthy rehabilitation. But be patient and follow the advice of your doctor or therapist. Returning to activity too soon, or not following the rehabilitation prescribed, can lead to long term problems.

Injury prevention

There are many steps that can be taken to prevent injuries occurring in the first place.

Ensure you have the appropriate equipment for a sport or activity – properly designed shoes, for example. It is important to progressively, rather than suddenly, increase the intensity of workouts - many people make the mistake of starting enthusiastically but overdoing things, before technique has been mastered and the body has had chance to adjust.

Ensure you warm up before a workout, and cool down and stretch afterwards. Focus on stretching any areas of tightness – and only use stretches that you understand, or have been shown by a fitness professional.

Areas of weakness can be improved by specific exercises, stretches and techniques – e.g., resistance band work to strengthen the rotator cuff of the shoulder (a common site for injuries), foam rolling for hip flexor tightness. These can be performed before workouts, and also between them.

Regular sports massage or osteopathy will help to ensure muscles are appropriately aligned, with fewer areas of tension. This is particularly beneficial for people who exercise frequently. Sports massage differs greatly from familiar relaxing massage, and may be quite uncomfortable, if there are areas requiring work.

Glucosamine and chondroitin is a popular supplement for joint protection, and for reduction of joint pain, although there is little scientific evidence for its efficacy.

Aches, pains and work

Office work is responsible for a wide range of musculoskeletal complaints. Prevent or reduce these with the following tips:

- Ensure you have the appropriate equipment – many offices discourage employees from spending long periods of time working at a laptop. A computer screen should be at eye level. You may also require a back support, foot rest and ergonomic equipment such as a trackball mouse

- Stretch regularly throughout the day
- Take regular breaks from the desk
- Drink plenty of water

Stretching and taking breaks is also important with other types of work, particularly physical jobs.

We tend to forget that there are muscles in the eye, controlling eye movements, the size of the pupil and the tension of the lens. Eye strain can cause headaches – book regular eye tests, and update spectacle prescriptions as necessary. If performing close work, every 15 minutes or so, make sure to change the point on which your eyes focus by looking at a distant object for a few seconds.

This summer, don't forget...

More of the body is on show during summer, and thinking about how to look one's best can also lead to health benefits. Consider the following:

Foot care

- Feet are often neglected, but keeping them healthy means they are more presentable in sandals, and foot care is an excellent long-term habit to maintain
- See your GP or a podiatrist if you have specific foot problems such as ingrowing toenails. Fungal infections of the nails and skin can be treated easily with over-the-counter products, and once cleared can be prevented by keeping feet dry. In some cases of fungal infection, removing yeast from the diet (bread, beer, wine) can resolve the problem entirely
- Remember that foot injuries can take longer to heal, so be kind to your feet with comfortable foot wear at least part of the time

The lymphatic system

- The lymphatic system is the little-discussed counterpart of the blood circulation – correct functioning is vital for health, and helps to reduce skin puffiness and the appearance of cellulite
- Encourage lymphatic flow with regular movement, skin brushing and hydration. When sitting for long periods, take regular breaks to engage the muscles

Chapter summary

- In June, consider how nutrition and fitness plans can be increased in intensity or otherwise modified - this might be the month to start restricting intake of certain types of food, or to trial a re-introduction
- Think about nutrient timing too - it may be possible to get more out of a gym session, or to feel more alert during the afternoon, by simply changing the times at which certain foods are eaten
- Be aware of the effect warmer weather can have on healthy lifestyle plans, and make sure yours is manageable for the summer months

Workbook section

Aspects of diet/lifestyle/fitness improvement I have made during the first half of the year:

What has made a difference:

What doesn't work for me:

Exercise – what I may need to change:

Nutrition – what I may need to change:

What I might need to address with a professional:

My thoughts on summer eating and exercise:

My hopes and intentions for the next half of the year:

July

Healthy holidays

Summer means increased leisure and holidays, and as the only time when outdoor celebration is possible, the summer months would have traditionally been the time for games, sports and other forms of enjoyment in England. However, they also involved hard work for agrarian communities, with weeding and protecting, and then the harvesting and sorting of crops.

The month in English is named for Julius Caesar, and in the Anglo-Saxon calendar its name means "after Litha". June was "before Litha", with Litha itself being midsummer. In some Slavic languages, the month's name is derived from natural phenomena. In Czech it is červenec, relating to redness, in Croatian, srpanj, meaning the sickle month (harvesting), in Polish it is lipiec, linden tree month (similarly in Ukrainian and Belarusian, it is lipen').

There are no specific public or church festivals during July, although there are individual saints' days, including the feasts of St Elijah on 20 July and of Mary Magdalene on 22 July. Perhaps this is because July represented intense work, and also due to a publically sanctioned reason to celebrate and relax not being required.

This month's chapter is focused on holidays, getting the best from the sun, and enjoying healthier breaks. Many people give up on healthy lifestyle initiatives over the summer, meaning these need to be started again, almost from scratch, in the autumn. Whilst summer should be about relaxation and enjoyment, retaining some degree of focus on nutrition and exercise throughout the warmer months will have immediate and longer term benefits, including improved energy levels and reduced risk of fat gain. Additionally, maintaining a healthier lifestyle is easier during summer in many respects - lighter food is appealing, exercise feels natural and work schedules are often reduced, so capitalise on this and you may see great results that you will want to maintain during autumn and winter.

Time in the sun

The dangers of exposure to the sun's rays are frequently emphasised, but the importance of sunlight for health should not be forgotten. UV radiation is required for the natural production of vitamin D, an essential hormone which is important for bone and cardiovascular health, immune system regulation and cancer prevention (see October chapter), and exposure to sunlight may have beneficial effects on mood.

Skin cancers and ageing

There are 3 main forms of skin cancer, derived from different skin cells:

- Basal cell carcinoma is the most common skin cancer,and comes from the basal (bottom) cells of the epidermis. It occurs on sun-exposed areas of skin, such as the face, ears and hands. Basal cell carcinomas are easily identified and can be cured, but can become more invasive if left untreated
- Squamous cell carcinoma, the second most common type of skin cancer, arises from the so called "scale-like" cells in the upper epidermis. The first step in the development of this cancer is actinic keratosis, patches of discolouration. Both actinic keratoses and squamous cell carcinoma are easily identified, as they occur on sun exposed areas of skin, such as the face and hands, and can be cured with treatment. A small percentage can become disfiguring, and a tiny proportion, if left without treatment, can be life-threatening
- Melanoma, from the pigment-bearing melanocytes is the

rarest and most dangerous form of skin cancer. Melanomas occur most commonly on the back, arms and legs, but do not occur only on sun exposed parts of the body – they can occur inside the mouth, on the vulva and in the back of the eye. There are four subtypes of melanoma – superficial spreading melanoma, nodular melanoma, acral lentiginous melanoma (which occurs on the soles of the foot and palms of the hand) and lentigi maligna melanoma (occurs on heavily sun damaged skin, usually less dangerous than the other types)

The first two types of skin cancer are common, and are related to cumulative exposure to UV – meaning that people who frequently spend time in the sun throughout their lives are at greatest risk. They are very rarely fatal, and affect mostly elderly people.

Malignant melanoma can be fatal, and can affect young people. Having numerous episodes of blistering sunburn, particularly during childhood, is a risk factor for developing melanoma, but asserting that sun exposure of any kind increases risk for the cancer may be simplistic, especially given that the cancer can form in areas not exposed to sun. Indeed, the most common areas for melanoma development are not the parts of the body such as the face and hands, which are habitually exposed to the sun. Other risk factors for melanoma include fair skin type, family and personal history, as well obesity and number of atypical moles on the skin. Use of sunbeds also carries a small increase in the risk of melanoma.

If you sunbathe regularly now, or did so in the past, or have used sunbeds, book in for a mole check - these are available on the high street, as well as through private medical clinics. Moles (beauty spots, freckles) are areas of increased pigmentation on the skin, and most are completely harmless. They can be flat or raised, and can vary in colour from pink to black, but should be checked regularly - changes in moles can relate to melanoma. Some individuals naturally have more pigmented spots than others, but if you have a large number of moles, sunbed use must be avoided and you should take extra care in the sun.

Monitor moles on a regular basis, looking out for ABCDE:

- Asymmetry - normal moles are most often symmetrical (i.e. a regular shape)
- Their Borders, which should be well defined
- Colour - moles can be a variety of colours in a given individual, but a mole should contain one colour only
- Diameter - normal moles tend to be smaller than 6mm across
- Evolution - any changes to the size, shape or condition of a mole. Bleeding and weeping are warning signs. New moles should also be checked

Some clinics offer photographic services to allow customers to keep a record of moles on the back.

Daily use of sunscreen is encouraged, even on cloudy days in the UK, although concerns have been raised over the safety of sunscreens. Many formulations contain substances such as oxybenzone, a synthetic oestrogen, and titanium dioxide, which are thought to increase levels of DNA-damaging free radicals. There is now a limit for the amount of oxybezone that can be included in a sunscreen. The Environmental Working Group suggests that whilst sunscreens do prevent sunburn, when used alone they do not reduce the risk of skin cancer.

Sunscreens do have their uses, and formulations with fewer potentially harmful chemicals are available. Rather than relying entirely sunscreens, though, it may be advisable to seek shade, cover up and use a hat.

The pattern of skin exposure seen in many British people today may be particularly conducive to melanoma development

– avoidance of the sun for much of the year (because sunlight levels are low in the UK and much of the population has an indoor lifestyle), and then intense exposure in a hot country for a few weeks.

Apart from the role of sun exposure in causation of skin cancers, UV exposure does contribute significantly to ageing of the skin. Moisturisation and adequate intake of antioxidants can help to combat this, but if premature skin ageing is a concern, sun exposure should be minimised, and a vitamin D3 supplement taken.

Our relationship with the sun

The sun is necessary to life on Earth, and exposure to sunlight has important benefits. Humans have had a relationship with the sun for thousands of years, worshipping it and following and celebrating its stations with festivals. No doubt there was also an element of respect and knowledge in this – understanding that hot weather can dry up sources of water, scorch crops and exhaust animals and humans. Now that relationship is becoming lost, and sunlight is seen as a danger, almost in the same class as cigarettes for its potential to damage health, or merely as a cosmetic aid.

Heavy use of sunscreens and beliefs about sun exposure may be contributing to the lack of connection between human behaviour and the sun. Where sunscreen is less routinely used, for example in rural communities in East and South East Asia, ways to reduce exposure to the sun have been developed, for example, wearing wide hats whilst working outdoors. In the warmer climates of Southern Europe, businesses typically close for several hours around midday, and the hottest hours of the day are given over to rest and avoiding the sun. Avoiding or limiting sun exposure is encouraged in very hot countries, the perceived attractiveness of a fair complexion in such countries attests to this.

In the UK, the opposite is true – despite multiple health warnings, a tanned look remains in fashion, and sunbeds and self tanning products are popular, due to our unpredictable climate.

Given the importance of vitamin D, the role of sunlight exposure in setting circadian rhythms and in improving mood, it is not surprising that people living in temperate climates would have generally taken every opportunity to enjoy the sun. In spring, the sun's rays are weaker, but skin is fairer, after the winter. Vitamin D is synthesised more quickly in pale skin, and so only relatively small exposures would have been required to produce it. As the weather improves, the amount of vitamin D that can be made through exposure increases, but so does the potential for damage, requiring a darkening of the skin. By the end of summer, darker skin requiring longer or more intense sun exposure to produce vitamin D results, but this darker skin is also better protected from the potential for damage. It is not possible to tell whether this system evolved in order to maximise vitamin D production, or by chance, but in any case there does seem to be a correlation between human behaviour, physiology and the relative intensity of the sun's rays.

The current practice of fair-skinned northern Europeans with no prior sun exposure spending hours in the intense sun of a tropical country, "protected" by chemicals, should perhaps be re-evaluated, and a healthier relationship with the sun developed.

Sun safety summary

- Avoid burning, through a combination of preventing over-exposure, covering up and using sunscreen. Sunscreen may be particularly useful when playing sport – look out for brands that are free of oxybenzone if you are concerned about the risks of this chemical. The same recommendations apply to children – extra care will need to be taken to ensure skin remains adequately covered

- Depending on your skin type and the season, regular sun exposure in the UK may have more benefits than risks. Exposing pale skin to the sun during a 30 degree heatwave will result in sunburn, and therefore skin damage and an increased risk of skin melanoma – whether this takes place in the UK or abroad, but regular, controlled exposure throughout the year could allow the skin to adapt, and would provide vitamin D, as well as boosting mood
- Remember that the amount of sun exposure that is safe for an individual depends on a variety of factors, including skin type, family history, number of moles, and the strength of the sun. In countries such as Australia, where fair skinned people spend a large amount of time in intense sun, melanoma rates are high. If you are unsure as to how much sun exposure is safe for you, always err on the side of caution, cover up and increase exposure gradually, to prevent burning
- Sunbeds may have a role in stimulating vitamin D synthesis in severely deficient adults who cannot tolerate supplements and who live in climates with little sun, but should not be used with the aim of getting a tan, because of the increase in the risk of melanoma, and should be avoided by children and teenagers. There is equipment available that produces visible light and the less damaging frequencies of UV, which is purported to have all the beneficial effects of sunlight without any of the risks, and use of this would be preferable to sunbeds (although it is much less widely available - see Resources section)
- Keep skin moisturised, and ensure an adequate intake of antioxidants from vegetables and fruit to help limit skin damage

- If preventing skin ageing is particularly important to you, reduce your exposure to the sun, and take a vitamin D supplement. The effects of the various chemicals used in cosmetics and sunscreen on skin ageing are not fully determined, so perhaps choose natural products and use sun avoidance. Skin ageing is also affected by pollution, smoking and other lifestyle factors, so a comprehensive approach is most effective
- Monitor moles on your skin, and see your doctor or a specialist if you are concerned about changes or new moles. If you have sunbathed extensively in the past, have used sunbeds, or have a large number of moles, book in a full mole check, and consider doing this regularly

Sun worship traditions

Changes in the seasons were marked in many cultures with festivals and rituals, suggesting the importance of the position of the sun. Use of fire in these rituals was common, and whilst fire will have had a practical purpose, symbolic associations are also likely.

A sun god featured in many cultures throughout the world. Sun deities were central to ancient Egyptian religion, with the sun god Ra being an important member of the pantheon. Other deities, such as the warrior goddess Sekhmet, were also connected with the sun, and there was a period of monotheistic worship of the sun disk Aten during the reign of the pharaoh Akhenaten (whose name incorporates that of the deity).

In Greek and Roman mythologies, the sun was associated with the male figures of Helios (Titan) and Apollo respectively. In Germanic and Norse mythology, the sun was represented by a goddess, Sol, and in Germanic languages, including English, the 7th day of the week is named for the sun. The Slavs may have venerated Dazhbog or Hors (in Eastern Slavic areas) as sun deities.

The role of the sun in the ancient pagan religions of the British Isles is unclear. Monuments such as Stonehenge may have been built in line with the path of the sun, although there is no evidence for sun veneration being their main purpose. Celts in Ireland and Wales did celebrate the opening of the seasons, and whilst this relates to the position of the sun, practical aspects related to farming were probably more important. The opening of the spring season on 1 February may have meant the start of sowing work in the fields, 1 May with the change to weeding and tending the crops, 1 August with the main bulk of the harvest and 1 November with the last harvests and preparation for winter. However, it is thought that the midwinter celebrations seen in many ancient cultures, including Roman and Anglo-Saxon Britain, are related to the "rebirth" of the sun.

Healthy holidays

Holidays are of course an opportunity for relaxation, and whilst a few weeks' indulgence would not usually undo months of hard work in the physical sense, breaking habits completely can mean they are difficult to resume, particularly post-holiday when low mood is common. Answer the following questions and find out how you can make your holidays healthier, whether you holiday at home or abroad.

What is the main reason for your holidays?

a) Escape, a break from everyday life, a chance to switch off
b) New cultural experiences
c) New experiences in the natural world, or adventure
d) Habit

It is difficult to maintain a diet and lifestyle routine on holiday where the main purpose of the holiday is escape. Any intrusion from "normal life" is likely to be resented. In this situation, consider why you feel the need to escape, and how your lifestyle can be modified to make taking a break less essential.

Where you want to take space from a job or a relationship, but are comfortable with your way of eating and exercise routine, try to separate food and exercise from other elements of daily life, and continue to eat well and stay active whilst on holiday. This does not mean daily gym attendance, or restricting food choices excessively – try other forms of activity, such as swimming, and enjoy the local cuisine without indulging daily in large amounts of alcohol, desserts or pasta, for example.

A diet and lifestyle that supports health should not be punishing or boring, and so plans that feel like a chore should be re-evaluated. It may, for example, be preferable to add small portions of whole grains, legumes and fruit to a strict low carbohydrate diet, to remove the "forbidden" label of such foods and provide more variety.

What sort of holidays do you usually choose?

a) Beach/pool based holidays in warm climates
b) Active or adventure holidays, such as camping or walking
c) Holidays where I can explore new cities and cultures
d) I like my holidays to be a mixture – some activity, some exploration some relaxation on the beach or by the pool

If you usually have an active holiday, with plenty of physical activity, then maintaining healthy habits will come naturally. Taking holidays focused on the pool or beach, or around cultural experiences may require more of an effort regarding activity:

- If out and about during the day, whether exploring a city or at the beach, make sure to have a protein-based breakfast. This will provide satiety during the morning
- Keep snacks such as fruit and nuts with you, to avoid snacking on ice creams, sandwiches and sweets

- If on a pool/beach holiday, build in time for activity every day – this does not have to be focused, progressive training. Consider using the hotel gym, or spending 15-20 minutes each evening on body weight exercises in your room. Swimming, long walks on the beach and in the surrounding areas, hiring a pedalo or canoe are all other ways to make activity part of your holiday

How do you arrange your meals on holiday?

a) I have an all-inclusive stay
b) I have breakfast at the hotel, and other meals in restaurants
c) I tend to self-cater
d) I have a mixture of self-catering and eating at cafes and restaurants

Self-catering for at least part of the holiday allows greater control over meals, and also provides an opportunity to cook with fresh local ingredients. Whatever form of meal provision you choose, try to avoid indulgent meals every day – after a particularly calorie-rich day, choose salads or vegetables, protein and small amounts of whole grains. All-inclusive stays in particular provide great scope for over-eating. Eat only as much as you need – not as much is available, adapt food intake to activity level and make a point of choosing salads and good quality lean protein as often as possible (taking care with cheese and dressings)

Does your alcohol intake increase on holiday?

a) Usually, yes
b) Not really

Drinking too much alcohol is common on holiday – local wines may be available, or exotic cocktails. A cold beer is also enticing on hot days, and all-inclusive deals make alcohol particularly accessible. Paying attention to alcohol consumption on holiday can minimise fat gain caused by the negative metabolic effects of the alcohol itself, and through the poor food choices often made whilst under the influence of alcohol. Setting a limit for alcohol, alternating alcohol drinks with water and drinking only at meals can all encourage healthy alcohol consumption patterns.

What about fruit?

The consumption of 5 portions of fruit or vegetables every day is encouraged, and the fibre, vitamins and antioxidants in fruit mean it is considered a healthy food. However, for fat loss, too much sugary fruit should be avoided. Fruit sugar, fructose, does not strongly impact insulin, but is processed in the liver. Any excess, not required for immediate conversion to glucose is stored as fat.

Some fruits such as apples, berries and sour cherries, are less sugary than others, and can be eaten more frequently, but swapping fruit for vegetables and salads can be helpful for fat loss.

The idea of fruit being a healthy breakfast is erroneous, as it does not provide a lasting source of energy. Fruit juices and smoothies are sources of concentrated fruit sugar and should be avoided.

On holiday in warmer climates, fresh fruits are more readily available, and these can be enjoyed daily in small amounts.

Should I take my supplements on holiday?

Supplements taken for a specific symptom or functional imbalance, such as low thyroid, adrenal insufficiency, or an imbalance in female hormones should be continued whilst on holiday. The same is true for supplements taken to correct a deficiency, such as iron, although it should be possible to leave vitamin D3 supplements at home if travelling to a sunny climate.

Certain supplements, such as fish oil liquid, flaxseed oil and many probiotics require refrigeration, and so should not be transported, although fish oil capsules do not usually require refrigeration. Omega-3 supplements are useful for supporting the skin whilst on holiday, and probiotics may be helpful for avoiding digestive upsets (see below).

With other supplements, taken for general support or to help manage stress, it is a matter of choice. Stress-relieving supplements, or those taken to help improve sleep may not be required on holiday, and a break in use may enhance their effectiveness.

If your goal is building muscle or increasing strength, you can continue to take a protein shake after intense workouts, if you work out on holiday. You may prefer to take portions of your own protein product with you, but provided you ensure you eat soon after training, a few weeks without protein shakes will not have a large effect. Protein shakes are not required after gentle workouts, at home, or abroad.

Antioxidants can help protect the skin from free radical damage, so ensure an adequate intake on holiday from vegetables, rather than expensive antioxidant supplements, which have been shown to be less effective.

Avoiding ill health on holiday

Going abroad can bring extra health risks, so speak to your doctor before travelling. You may be advised to take malaria prophylaxis, or to have certain vaccinations – some of these are required a few weeks in advance. Concerns have been raised about the safety of some vaccines, but discuss the risks and benefits with your doctor.

There are a variety of health problems that can adversely affect your holiday. Consider the following and make the most of your time away.

- Awareness starts on the plane – if taking a long haul flight, move regularly, and consider compression stockings and in some cases aspirin (check it is not contraindicated – it can cause Reyes syndrome in children). Eat lightly and stay hydrated
- There are a variety of travel sickness pills and products available, including homeopathic varieties and bracelets that work on pressure points. Fresh ginger is a natural and simple alternative
- Limit the impact of jet lag. Try to adjust your routine as soon as possible to your destination. If you arrive during the day, after a short rest (no more than a few hours), exercise gently and spend some time in the sun. The light and movement will help to re-set the circadian rhythm. If your destination is not sunny, consider using a portable SAD lamp (see October)
- Digestive upsets are common when travelling. Avoid local tap water, drinks with ice, salads and fruit, as well as undercooked meat. On long haul flights, do not accept drinks with ice, as local water from refuelling stops may have been used. Probiotic supplements may be helpful in protecting the floral balance of the intestine
- Pack oral rehydration salts in case of severe diarrhoea or vomiting. If you do develop an illness on holiday, seek medical advice
- Other essentials to pack include alcohol wipes and gel (wipes are useful for disinfecting cuts and grazes, gel can be used to disinfect hands), plasters, eye wash solution, antihistamine tablets and painkillers
- Holiday romances can end badly – it is thought that a sizeable minority of British holidaymakers return home with a sexually transmitted disease. Be cautious and stay safe – condoms may be another holiday essential
- In hotter climates dehydration can occur easily – stay

hydrated with water, and limit your intake of caffeine and alcohol

- Invest in travel insurance and ensure all other documentation (such as European Health Insurance Card) is in order. Find out in advance where medical help can be accessed

Chapter summary

- Enjoy a healthier holiday this summer - keeping alcohol intake in check, interspersing indulgent meals with lighter foods, and remaining active will mean you make the most of your break, looking and feeling your best
- Be sensible in the sun - regular, controlled exposure throughout the year may be helpful for maintaining vitamin D levels, but sudden exposure of pale skin to hot sun is likely to lead to sunburn
- Choose summer fruits wisely - fruits are rich in sugar, which can be stored as fat if not required immediately for energy. Fibrous and more sour fruits are the best options

Workbook section

What usually happens on holiday in terms of diet and lifestyle:

How this affects me:

What I plan to do differently this year:

Holiday notes:

Autumn

Completion
Drawing in
Re-evaluating

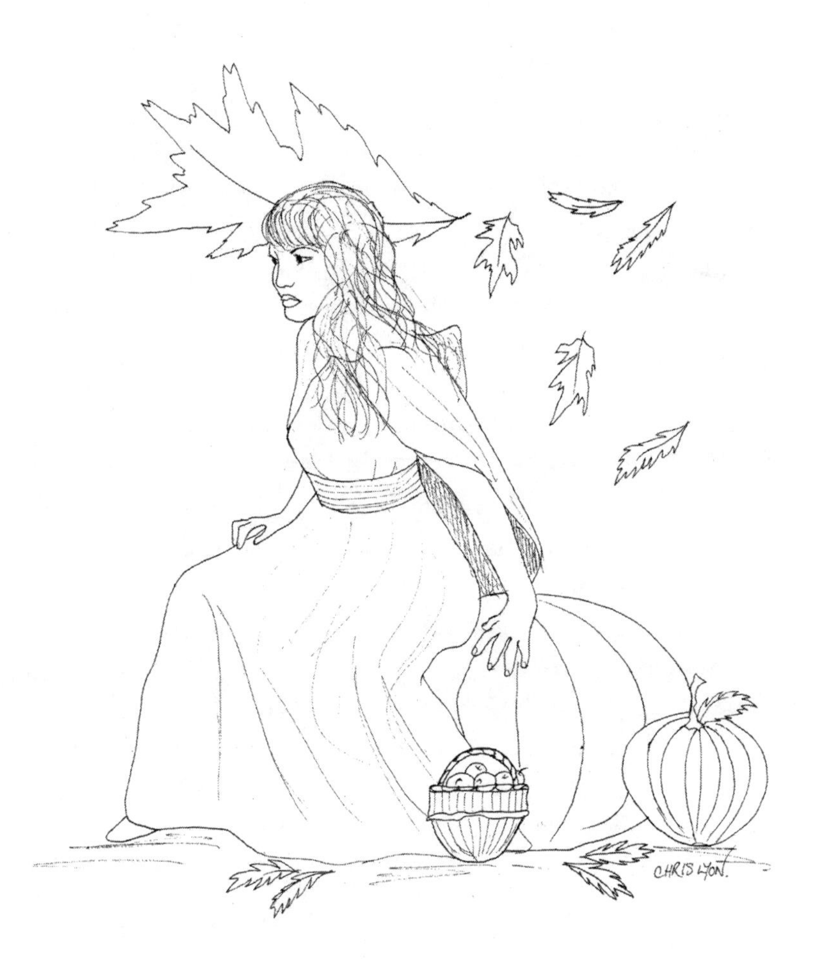

August

Mellowing of the season

August used to be considered the start of the English autumn season. Whilst some of the warmest days can occur now, the days begin to shorten, and occasionally there is the feeling that summer has passed its peak and that its energy is transforming.

Until the 19th century, much of the harvest took place during August in England, as would have been the case in other European countries (the month names in Czech, Croatian, Ukrainian, Belarusian and Polish all involve aspects of harvest). Subsequently, harvest activities also took place in July and September.

Harvest-related festivals took place in early August in Britain and Ireland, including the Celtic Lughnasa, in honour of the god Lugh (confusingly, not a harvest god), celebrated mainly in Ireland, and the separate Anglo-Saxon festival of "Loaf Mass" (Lammas) celebrated in England. At Lammas, the fruits of the first cereal harvest were baked and used as an offering to make the grain storage barn safe. It is possible that the Anglo-Saxon festival was adapted from the Celts, as a harvest celebration on 1 August is particular to England, and not found in other northern European countries. In any case, Lammas was important in England for centuries, being an occasion for a range of community and business activities.

Bringing in the crops involved hard physical labour, but also celebration - when not working in the fields, labourers would be found eating and drinking heartily, often at the expense of the farmer whose crops they were working on, and the time of year was generally popular for feasts, fairs and games, known as "wakes", "revels" or "hoppings", as well as for church dedication celebrations.

Particular importance was attached to bringing home the last sheaf of cereal. Legends arose about the magical properties of the last sheaf, and teams of labourers who had completed their harvest would taunt those from neighbouring farms with crops still standing. The significance of these activities decreased with advances in agricultural technology.

In the past, August would have meant working hard, playing hard and considering the outcome of months of labour. Today it is a relaxed month, corresponding to school and university holidays and a slower pace of activity for many businesses. The mellowing of the season makes it an appropriate month to think about dealing with stress, and the associations with harvest mean seasonal and local eating can be consider now.

Cortisol, the stress hormone, and its effects

Cortisol is one of the "fight or flight" hormones released by the small endocrine glands situated on top of the kidneys (adrenal glands), in response to stress. There are a range of glucocorticoid hormones which have a similar effect to cortisol, but the discussion here will focus on "cortisol" as a representative of the group.

Throughout most of human evolution, "stress" would have largely meant a pressure to flee, fight or expend significant effort – for example, hunting or being hunted, confronting or being confronted.

Cortisol has a less dramatic, but longer lasting effect than adrenaline, and its effects are directed towards preparation to fight or flee, including:

- Converting muscle amino acids into glucose, for immediate use by the brain and muscles
- Raising blood pressure to ensure blood reaches the muscles and brain
- Shutting down processes that are not essential to escaping, catching the prey or fighting, such as immune

system responsiveness, fertility, urination, storage of nutrients

Cortisol is an important hormone – absence or very low levels can be life threatening. Conversely, excessively high levels of the hormone can lead to:

- Fat storage in the abdominal area, particularly around the organs
- Increased risk of heart disease
- Depression, and problems with cognition and memory
- Thyroid imbalances
- Thinning of the skin and bones, and loss of muscle mass
- Immune system suppression
- Menstrual irregularities in women
- Reduced libido

High levels of cortisol are common amongst people living in industrialised countries, as modern life means that instead of being stimulated occasionally, in response to temporary threats, the cortisol system is stimulated every day, by ever-present stressors.

Constant demand on the adrenal glands to release cortisol can lead to their exhaustion and the condition known as adrenal fatigue (see February chapter). A person at risk of adrenal exhaustion may feel constantly "wired" – stressed, anxious and unable to relax, with poor sleep. As the adrenal function is compromised, this leads to a "tired but wired" feeling, with anxiety, stress and lethargy all coexisting. The final stage is physical and mental exhaustion.

There are a number of ways that the cortisol system can be modified. It is possible to reduce the amount of cortisol released from the adrenal glands, by affecting the hormones that stimulate these glands, as well as manipulating the proportion of cortisol that is free to interact with cells (rather than being bound to a transport protein). Finally, the enzyme 11-beta-hydroxysteroid-dehydrogenase-1 (HSD) amplifies the actions of cortisol within cells – so regardless of blood levels, it is possible to experience exaggerated stress hormone effects if HSD levels are high (such a situation is associated with obesity and insulin resistance). Conversely, reducing HSD levels can decrease the impact of cortisol.

Cortisol release normally has a circadian rhythm, with levels being higher in the morning and decreasing throughout the day. Low levels in the evening should correspond to a relaxed state, and disturbed secretion rhythms are a feature of adrenal fatigue – later stages of the condition involve no variation in cortisol levels. Therefore, many blood tests have little value in diagnosing adrenal fatigue – firstly because cortisol usually has a diurnal variation, and tests usually involve a single sample, and secondly, because in advanced adrenal fatigue, no variation is likely.

There are interactions and relationships between all hormones – cortisol and testosterone, for example, have the same precursor, and high levels of cortisol often mean low levels of testosterone – testosterone has a wide range of effects, including increasing bone and muscle mass, improving mood, increasing drive and increasing the rate of production of red blood cells and so it is important to support testosterone levels in both men and women.

Stress, mind/body duality and depression

Whether the stress response is considered in terms of hormones, or more generally, there is now sufficient evidence for certain forms of stress being an important factor in the development of a range of diseases, including heart disease, dementia, cancer, osteoporosis, stomach and duodenal ulcers, diabetes and depression. Whilst the term "stress" is generally used to mean "stress with negative impacts", positive forms of stress, which can be motivating, also exist. Adverse stress detrimentally affects sleep, sex drive, immunity and fertility and leads to fat gain.

Managing (detrimental) stress and balancing cortisol is therefore crucial for health and wellbeing, and this requires an awareness of the connection between body and mind. These two aspects of ourselves are generally considered to be separate, a world view promoted by the philosopher Descartes.

A growing body of work now suggests that mental and physical states are connected. Moods and cognition are modulated by neurotransmitters and hormones, and receptors for certain messenger substances are found both inside and outside the brain.

An important illness where body and mind can be seen to interact is depression. Both psychological and biochemical approaches to depression exist, but for those suffering from depression, a combined approach may be the most effective.

Clinical depression is more than sadness or a lack of optimism. In addition to low mood, depressed individuals gain little or no enjoyment from previously enjoyable activities and experience disturbance in their sleeping and eating patterns. They may also experience feelings of worthlessness and hopelessness, and become unable to function socially or at work. Sometimes a negative life event can trigger clinical depression, but there is not always a "reason" for depression.

Unipolar depression, with the symptoms described above, should be distinguished from bipolar affective disorder (manic depression). As well as periods of low mood, lethargy and hopelessness, individuals with bipolar affective disorder also experience periods with increased activity levels, reduced need for food or sleep and overactive mental processes. A bipolar individual in the manic phase may be exceptionally creative, and/or destructive.

There are many hypotheses as to the cause of the different

types of depression, but the prevailing view in the last few decades has been that deficiency of the neurotransmitter (brain chemical required for conduction of nerve impulses) serotonin , and similar substances is the main cause of unipolar depression. Correcting the deficiency with drugs that increase the concentration of serotonin is believed to be the best the way to solve the problem, implying that thoughts and feelings can be easily modified with chemicals.

Widespread use of drugs that affect the serotonin system (Serotonin Specific Reuptake Inhibitors and Serotonin and Noradrenaline Reuptake Inhibitors) has its disadvantages – these drugs can have significant side effects, including increased risk of suicide ideation in young people, sexual dysfunction, headaches, dizziness, gastrointestinal disturbance and bone marrow suppression.

Serotonin and noradrenaline are not the only body chemicals associated with depression – high levels of cortisol may also be implicated in the disease, and so dealing with the neurotransmitters alone, and not looking at hormones and other aspects of the body, may not provide a complete solution.

Some schools of thought focus more on psychological approaches to the treatment of depression, and there are many talking therapy approaches including counselling, psychotherapy and Cognitive-Behavioural Therapy (CBT). CBT is the best researched, and the most widely promoted within the medical profession, but criticisms as to its longer-term effectiveness do exist. It is attractive as rather than involving lengthy sessions analysing the childhood causes of particular behaviours or thinking patterns, it is practical and outcome-focused. This may be a weakness of the method, as well as a strength. Practising more constructive thinking patterns may be helpful in the shorter term, but if underlying issues are not addressed, problems may re-surface. Cognitive-Analytical Therapy can be thought of as combining aspects of CBT and analysis/

psychotherapy.

If you feel low in mood and have noticed changes in your sleeping or eating patterns, or if you find it difficult to find enjoyment in life, speak to your doctor. Be sure to discuss all the options, including talking therapies and lifestyle modification. Whilst prescription drugs do help many people with depression, particularly when used for a short period, to allow the person to function more effectively and take other forms of action, the causes of depression are more complex than a deficiency in one or two neurotransmitters.

See the October chapter for a discussion of seasonal depression – many of the therapies with proven efficacy for seasonal depression are also helpful for forms of depression that do not vary with the time of year. If you suffer strongly from SAD, you might wish to start light therapy as early as August, as light levels are already beginning to decline.

Managing stress, balancing cortisol

There are a number of ways to approach balancing cortisol:

- Reducing or modifying the stimuli for cortisol release (reducing "stress")
- Helping the body to better deal with stressful stimuli
- Helping the body to better deal with cortisol and other hormones

Reducing or modifying the stimuli for cortisol release

Fluctuating levels of sugar and insulin lead to fluctuations of cortisol, so avoiding refined and processed foods will go some way to stabilising both insulin and cortisol – modifying the diet is one of the first steps that can be taken to improve cortisol balance.

Reducing negative psychological stress is key to reducing the negative effects of cortisol and could involve identifying specific stressors and then developing an action plan. Use the workbook section at the end of this chapter as a guide for identifying specific areas for attention.

Helping the body to better deal with stressful stimuli

It is not possible to avoid all stressful stimuli, but the way in which these are dealt with can nearly always be improved. Neuro-Linguistic Programming or reframing techniques may be helpful here.

Regular, moderate exercise allows the diversion of the fight/flight response into physical activity, and exercise is a helpful release for those with stressful schedules - although excessive exercise is a form of stress and increases cortisol release; with some forms of exercise being particularly conducive to cortisol system stimulation. A common mistake made by people affected by stress-related fat gain is to devote themselves to long duration, low intensity exercises, such as jogging, in the hope that this will burn fat – such activity is more likely to damage joints and increase cortisol levels, meaning more efficient fat storage.

Another approach to dealing with stressful stimuli involves actively relaxing – activities such as Tai Chi, massage and walking are ideal, but it does not always feel possible to set aside large chunks of time, even though doing so can create increased efficiency. The following list suggests some quick ways to relax, and one universal pointer is to try avoiding the use of food or alcohol as regular ways to manage stress.

You might find some of the following helpful:

- Reading a book or magazine, even if just for 15 minutes – this takes attention away from the stressful situation
- Meditation – focusing on your breathing is an easy way to start

- Spending time with plants or animals
- Painting, drawing, doodling
- Performing some simple stretches – releasing muscle tension can have knock-on effects on mental tension
- Catching up with friends
- Drinking a relaxing herbal blend of tea
- Helping others, e.g., voluntary work
- Using the sauna or steam room

Helping the body to better deal with cortisol and other hormones
Ensuring general good nutrition will provide the body with the vitamins, minerals and other cofactors required to effectively balance cortisol. In addition, certain supplements are recommended specifically for cortisol and testosterone balance, and for the control of HSD. Some of these, such as phosphatidylserine and theanine, are also useful for improving sleep (see April chapter)

Herbs such as cordyceps, ginseng, Siberian ginseng, ashwaghanda, rhodiola, astragalus and holy basil have been used in Eastern medicine for centuries to improve vitality, boost immunity and help adaptation to stressful situations (hence the name "adaptogen"). Research has been carried out on the chemical components of the herbs and there have been some positive results in terms of the effects of the herbs on humans, such as:

- A blend of adaptogens including rhodiola rosea, schisandra and Siberian ginseng increased human cognitive performance under stress
- A randomised, controlled trial showed that rhodiola rosea extract improved symptoms of stress related fatigue and decreased cortisol response in humans
- Treatment with powdered ashwagandha root caused an improvement in semen parameters in infertile human males

Adaptogenic herbs may be helpful as part of an anti-stress plan. Whilst these herbs have a long history of use, backed up to a degree by research, there are many "miracle" claims attached to them. It is better to add an adaptogen to an anti-stress plan that also includes a sensible diet, adequate sleep and exercise, rather than expecting a new lease of life from a supplement. Consulting a herbalist or naturopath may also help in identifying which adaptogen would be best suited to you.

The importance of friends and neighbours for health

Despite communication being easier than ever, with an ever-growing list of ways to "stay in touch" and share information, modern life, particularly in cities, can be lonely. It is no longer common for several generations of a family to cohabit, or even to live near to one another, family units are decreasing in size and generally, the whole concept of the family has declined in importance in many western countries. The demands of the typical work schedule mean it can even be difficult to maintain meaningful contact with close friends, and since religion plays less of a part in today's society, yet another arena for building relationships has been lost. Large numbers of people live alone, and much socialisation may take place with work colleagues or acquaintances.

The impact this situation may have on health has largely been ignored, although a study in July 2010 (published in PLoS Medicine) showed that people with strong social networks are more likely to live longer. This correlates with observations made on the town of Roseto in the US. The town's population came almost exclusively from a town of the same name in Italy, and was modelled closely on its namesake. Researchers were surprised to find that cardiovascular mortality was a fraction of that of a neighbouring town, despite high levels of obesity and a diet rich in foods generally connected with poor cardiovascular health. The difference was attributed to strong, southern

European style social networks.

Being with other people can be an effective way to deal with some forms of stress, and can also protect health. It may thus be worth making sure that in the whirl of social media and text messages, real contact with friends is not lost, and that time is set aside to spend with family.

Scheme for dealing with stress and its impacts

1. See your doctor if stress is having a major effect on your life
2. Remove physiological stressors as much as possible – e.g., overindulgences in alcohol, convenience foods, overuse of caffeine, irregular meals, inadequate sleep
3. Decrease psychological stressors (using the table at the end of the chapter as a guide) – e.g., take steps to improve work/home situations
4. Introduce a healthy exercise regime – not over-exercising or focusing on long duration cardiovascular work. This does not have to involve joining a gym – it could begin with taking a brisk 30 minute walk every day
5. Actively relax, even if this is just 15 minutes before bed and introduce stress-relieving activities, which could range from yoga practice to regularly catching up with friends
6. Ensure an optimal balance of nutrients, which may involve taking some basic supplements
7. Consider introducing a herbal stress supplement or adaptogen. As well as raising the issue again with your doctor, seek advice from a naturopath, practitioner of Chinese Medicine or other complementary health professional, to ensure the herbal supplement regime is tailored appropriately to your needs

Seasonal food in England

Year-round availability of any type of food and the convenience of supermarkets are dominant factors in the shopping behaviours of most Britons. Factory farming and the growth of a food "industry" has made once exclusive foods commonplace, and previously commonplace occurrences, such as people growing their own foods, and enjoying the fruits of the season – have now become exclusive, limited to those who have the financial resources or the time to seek out or grow such produce.

Confused by the goods flown in from New Zealand, Thailand or Brazil, shoppers fail to appreciate the richness of the local harvests. August is an excellent month to enjoy seasonal berries, such as strawberries, raspberries, gooseberries and blackberries as well as peaches, broad beans, artichokes or courgettes, to name a few. The mass production of food has brought us convenience – long shelf lives and constant availability – and this, not taste, variety or quality, is what we consistently pay for in supermarkets. The ubiquity of processed food compounds the problem – few people would stop to think about the origin of the individual ingredients in a supermarket-bought sandwich.

Trying to cheat the seasons is nothing new, it was at the heart of the earliest agricultural methods, where grain could be harvested and used for food throughout the year. Many methods of preserving food, so it can be enjoyed out of season, are ancient, as is trade in exotic foods, Now though, eating unseasonal food is the normal situation for the majority of people, and knowledge of seasonality has been completely lost.

The seasonality of foods can be thought of as mirroring the health requirements of humans and other animals. Nutrient dense root vegetables are available in the winter, providing sustenance for the colder weather, and this is also the time when it is best to obtain and eat richer meats such as venison and goose. The abundance of leafy vegetables in the summer fits well with the requirement for a lighter diet rich in antioxidants, and the appearance of fruit at the end of summer and in autumn could even be thought of providing a tasty way to gain fat to last through the winter.

Seasonal, local food tastes better. Test this for yourself, noting the difference between an early English apple (such as Katy or Discovery), and a variety from the other side of the planet, or between in-season English tomatoes from a local farm or allotment, and a supermarket product, flown in from Europe. Eating seasonally and locally greatly benefits the environment and local producers, and can be more cost effective too. Whilst heirloom vegetables and rare breeds meat remain more expensive than supermarket fare, because of the effort required to produce them, more commonplace locally grown foods are often priced very competitively, since the cost of transport, storage and packaging is removed. To find seasonal and local foods, it is often necessary to shop at places other than supermarkets, although in August, a variety of local produce can be found even there.

Simple changes in shopping habits encourage us to slow down, build relationships with suppliers and develop a healthy focus on food, as well as fostering consideration of how to create a balanced meal, or of what else can be done with a particular crop of fruit or vegetables – rather than obsession over calories or grams of carbohydrate or fat. Food becomes a means of connection with the earth and with other people, and a way to express creativity, rather than fuel to grab whilst doing something else or a dangerous yet addictive substance that should be avoided as much as possible. Even if no effort is made to "diet", it is highly likely that a person living in Britain basing most meals on seasonally available British foods would soon lose weight and feel healthier.

Consider how you can eat more seasonally. See the Resources section for books and websites, but also consider:

- Regularly visiting farmers' markets or farm shops – not only will this allow you to buy good quality, fresh produce, but it will support the growth of a more sustainable food industry too. As such enterprises grow in popularity, they are becoming more accessible, with inner city availability of farm produce, and the expansion of rural farm shops
- Signing up for "fresh from the farm" delivery services, which can provide meat, fish, poultry vegetables, fruit and even prepared foods such as home made jam or bread. Some of these services provide excellent value for money
- Finding out where you can pick your own, seasonally
- Growing some of your own produce, in a garden, allotment or in small pots
- Trying out traditional recipes, such as for preserves and pickles (see the References section for books) – so that the abundance of summer can be of benefit during the winter

These steps may not be realistic for everyone, and it is possible to adapt supermarket shopping towards seasonal and local food. If supermarkets note a demand for local produce, and decrease in sales of air-freighted goods and convenience foods, they will adapt accordingly. Avoid obvious incongruities, such as strawberries or asparagus in winter, and when local produce is available in the supermarket, consider buying in bulk and freezing, or otherwise storing or preserving.

Chapter summary

- Make the most of a relaxed time of year to consider which relaxation methods work best for you, and plan to carry these on after the summer
- If your lifestyle is stressful, try to identify the specific problematic elements. It is also important to optimise

your diet and exercise routine, to minimise the effects of stress on your body

- August means an abundance of seasonal, local foods. Take the opportunity to find out how you can obtain them, and keep in mind how you can eat more seasonally and locally all year round

Workbook section

Areas of my life that currently cause me stress and affect me negatively, on a regular basis (E.g., work, relationship with partner, family members, my appearance, my financial situation)

Specific causes of stress in this area:

e.g., (Work) Often having to work long hours, depending on client demands

Simple short term steps I can take to reduce impact
e.g., Making sure I take regular breaks throughout the day, focusing on relaxation at weekends, decreasing use of alcohol as a means to relax in the evenings, as I often feel worse the next day

Medium term steps I can take to reduce impact
e.g., Discuss situation with boss, learn some stress relief techniques, take up a hobby so work is not such a focus

Longer term solutions
e.g., Change of career

How I can start eating more seasonally and locally:
Ideas for storing/preserving foods that are currently available, for use during the winter

September

Harvest home

Being called Holy Month by the Anglo Saxons, and containing the Autumn Solstice modern Harvest Festival celebrations and the start of the academic year, September is important for cultural events. The non-Latin names for this month translate as the shining month, the red month and the month of heather.

In ancient Rome, games were held in honour of Jupiter in September, and the feasts of Septimonium (relating to the number 7 and the 7 hills of Rome – September was the 7th month until the addition of July and August) and of Venus the mother were also celebrated in September. Modern-day Wiccans celebrate the feast of Mabon around the Autumn equinox, although there is no evidence for pre-Christian festivals around this date.

Michaelmas, the feast of St Michael the Archangel, patron saint of the sea falls on September 29. It was a church feast day until the reformation, and was celebrated for some time after that in the fishing communities of the outer Hebrides. The autumn term is still referred to as Michaelmas term at the University of Cambridge, but overall September is not now a month when large scale public festivals take place – most Harvest Festivals tend to be modest affairs, arranged by schools or churches, sometimes involving donations of food to the less fortunate.

A period of transition, September presents opportunities to take stock of your situation. It is also the month to start considering how you will prepare your body for the colder months ahead.

Taking stock and planning for the months ahead

The weather can still be reasonably warm and bright, but the harvest is home, and the changing colours of the landscape attest to the inevitable change of season. The twenty-first of September sees day and night being equal in length – thereafter, night begins to dominate.

September is a time for thoughtfulness, encouraged by the warm colours and mellow light. As trees shed their leaves, and the vibrant flowers of spring and summer draw inwards, into seeds and fruits for storage, think about discarding what no longer works and start to focus energy inwards. Use space at the end of the chapter for a progress review.

Whether a specific public event took place in early Autumn or not, it is likely that in the past, communities would have considered how best to prepare for the colder months ahead. A major feature may have been the preservation of foods gathered at the harvest. Now is the time to prepare for the rest of the year in terms of health, wellbeing and fitness.

Autumn can be beautiful, but it is often a season of coughs and colds, and of declining mood, as the nights begin to draw in. Mass returns to work, school and university are no doubt partially responsible for the increases in respiratory infections in autumn.

September may be a good month to start taking supplements, particularly for those who regularly experience ill health during the colder months.

Ensuring sufficient exposure to natural light, or a substitute, is important, as is ensuring your vitamin D levels are adequate – see October chapter for more on this topic.

Boosting the immune system

What is the immune system?

The immune system protects the body from negative influences. These include bacteria, viruses, parasites and internal threats such as cancer cells. It is a highly complex set of cells and processes, and includes barriers such as the skin and mucous membranes, and the fatty acids and antibodies found there, as well as the white blood cells and antibodies. The actions of the immune system have been recognised for thousands of years – when the immune system is activated by injury or infection, inflammation ensues, comprising redness, swelling heat and pain with loss of function.

A healthy immune system reacts only to threatening stimuli (pathogens), whilst ignoring others. This relies on the maintenance of a delicate balance of chemical signals between the different elements of the system. This is easily disturbed, and situations where the immune system reacts inappropriately and causes harm are common – hayfever and autoimmune diseases such as multiple sclerosis, hypothyroidism and type 1 diabetes are some examples. Inflammatory components are thought to exist in many chronic diseases, meaning that immune system balance may emerge as a key determinant of health.

The hygiene hypothesis has been put forward to explain the increases in allergies and autoimmune disorders seen in the developed world – a lack of exposure to infections, particularly from parasites, in childhood means that parts of the immune system are under-stimulated – resulting in hyperactivity of other parts of the system.

The immune system can be broadly classified into the innate immune system and the adaptive immune system. The innate immune system acts rapidly and is widely distributed through the body. Its cells engulf or destroy pathogens. The adaptive immune response, mediated by T and B cells, "learns" to recognise pathogens or pathogen-infected cells, and attacks them either through the use of specialised proteins (antibodies) or through disrupting cell membranes. Its purpose is to increase the effects of the innate immune system, and to detect pathogens not dealt with already.

Immune system regulation is still poorly understood, although vitamin D, protein intake, stress levels and micronutrient balance are thought to be important.

Preventing and dealing with coughs and colds

There are many natural ideas for supporting the immune system, and for preventing or relieving coughs and colds. Start with the basics – provide the body with the raw materials required for a healthy immune system, and reduce physiological stressors. Some supplements have been proven to reduce the frequency or severity of colds, but choose wisely, as there is a confusing array of so-called immune boosting products.

Diet

An adequate intake of protein from animal and/or vegetable sources is important for immune function, and vegetables provide vitamins, minerals and phytochemicals, as well as fibre, which allows the efficient elimination of waste products.

Cold foods such as salads become less appealing in autumn, and in some cultures, eating cold foods in colder weather is not advised. Cook vegetables lightly, and start to experiment with soups, casseroles and stews. Make the most of vegetables such as squashes and use spices to create warming, interesting dishes.

Consider minimising use of dairy products, as these can increase mucous congestion.

The following foods and ingredients have a reputation for being useful during the respiratory infection season:

Chicken soup

The purported healing properties of this dish are thought to have first been recorded by a rabbi in the 12th century – it is popular around the globe in various forms, and is thought to help recovery from respiratory infections, although there is no scientific evidence to support this.

Sage tea

Drinking sage tea to support the respiratory system and aid recovery from coughs and colds is popular in some European countries. No randomised controlled trials have been conducted with sage tea, but chemical components of the plant have been shown to have biological activity, killing bacteria in the laboratory setting.

Ginger

Spices are typical ingredients during autumn and winter, and ginger is used extensively against the force of cold in Chinese medicine, where "cold" has a specific meaning. It has different indications when used fresh or dried – fresh ginger is used to treat colds, flu, lung problems and sore throats, as well as digestive issues. The dried root is used for general coldness.

Feed a cold, starve a fever?

The old wives' tale that eating helps recovery from a cold, whereas fasting can help to reduce a fever may have an element of truth. In 2002, researchers found that meals stimulated the parts of the immune system that deal with viruses, and so could be helpful for colds, and that fasting stimulated other parts of the immune system, which work against bacteria. However, going without food for those unused to fasting is generally not advisable.

Exercise

Regular exercise is important for hormonal balance and for boosting energy levels, but overexertion should be guarded against during autumn and winter. This may involve a decrease in the number of sessions per week, or a change in the type of exercise performed. Intense training is a form of stress on the body, and can suppress the immune system if adequate opportunity for recovery is not taken between sessions. Do not train through a cold.

Lifestyle

Stress management

Cortisol has an immunosuppressive effect – analogues are used as therapies for autoimmune and allergic diseases, so minimising stress, and its effects on the body is particularly key during autumn - review the discussions in the August chapter.

Spa therapy

Alternating heat and cold are therapies are thought to be useful for strengthening the body against disease, and are popular in many cultures. Research has shown that sauna bathing may lower blood pressure, as well as decreasing the pain of musculoskeletal conditions.

Studies on cold water immersion, which often accompanies sauna bathing, have provided support for this practice. Regular immersions in cold water slightly increased the concentration of white blood cells in the blood of healthy young men. Thus, as well as supporting the immune system indirectly through stress management, spa therapies such as sauna/plunge and hot water bathing may provide a direct boost.

Supplements

There are many supplements claiming to boost the immune system – some of these do have a well reported effect, and are worth considering for the autumn and winter.

Vitamin C

Whilst there is little evidence for the effectiveness of mega-doses of vitamin C, particularly after a cold has started, research has shown that daily doses of the vitamin (500mg) can reduce cold frequency in some situations.

Verdict: Inexpensive, easy to obtain and effective in certain situations.

Vitamin D

When converted into its active hormonal form in the body, vitamin D is a powerful regulator of the immune system. Low levels of vitamin D within a population may help to spread respiratory infections.

Verdict: Vitamin D is important for many aspects of health. Supplements are easy to obtain and reasonably priced. Check for any contraindications and book a blood test to find out your vitamin D levels first.

Echinacea

Extracts of echinacea have become extremely popular for preventing colds, and research has shown that they can decrease frequency and duration of colds - although overall, results of studies are conflicting.

Verdict: Another easy to obtain, reasonably priced supplement with some support from studies. Worth a try if you tend to suffer from coughs and colds during autumn and winter.

Astragalus

Used in Chinese medicine for centuries, astragalus has been hailed as "the new echinacea", although there is little direct evidence for its usefulness against colds and flu.

Verdict: Used for hundreds of years, and research may point towards its effects on the immune system – but there is more evidence for echinacea as a herbal supplement to prevent colds.

Nasal sprays

Nasal sprays promoted as being able to stop colds from developing have become quite popular in the UK, but there is little scientific evidence for their efficacy. Saline sprays may be helpful for reducing feelings of congestion.

Verdict: Little evidence for efficacy of commercial products, and they can irritate the lining of the nose. Saline sprays may have a role in reducing congestion. Virucidal hand treatments may be of more use than "virus trapping" nasal sprays, particularly for people who spend long periods in contact with others, or who travel on public transport.

Glutamine

Glutamine is used widely by athletes and body builders to help recovery from training, and to support the immune system in demanding situations. It may help to repair the mucosa of the GI tract, and so could be a general supportive factor.

Verdict: Inexpensive and easy to obtain, and some of the anecdotal evidence is backed up by research.

Probiotics

Taking a good quality probiotic has been shown to reduce the severity and duration of respiratory infections, having effects in adults and children.

Verdict: Now may be the time to start using a probiotic supplement, but choose a brand which states its concentration.

Reishi mushroom

In China, reishi mushrooms have been used to treat a wide range of ailments for centuries. A mechanism of action has been proposed for their active compounds, but there is limited evidence for their ability to affect the immune system

Verdict: The claims are extravagant, and the mechanisms of action convincing, but as evidence is limited, perhaps only turn to this more expensive supplement if other approaches have not worked.

Grains

September, with its associations with the harvest, is a fitting month to think about grains.

For most of human existence, food was hunted and gathered, and humans lived in small groups, by necessity regularly changing location. Cultivation of wild grain species began in the Middle East around 10,000 years ago, where the climate was suited to the growth of large-seeded plants. It is thought that the conditions after the last Ice Age supported abundant growth of wild grasses, and that a subsequent cooler period then stimulated greater reliance on these as sources of food. A genetic mutation in an early form of wheat, causing seeds to remain on the stem after ripening, rather than dropping to the ground, may also have occurred, allowing seeds to be collected and stored for future sowing – automatically, such varieties of grass would have been favoured by early farmers, and would have eventually become dominant.

Over the millennia, increasing numbers of plants and animals were domesticated, and human populations became larger and more stable, leading to the development of towns and cities. Whilst agriculture enabled the development of human societies, it may also be responsible for familiar chronic diseases – remains of pre-agricultural humans are thought to demonstrate the superior health of these hunter-gatherers, compared with early town and city dwellers. Nevertheless, grains remained at the centre of the diet for many populations, as they could be grown in large quantities, stored, and also used as food for domesticated animals.

Wheat was an important food in ancient Egypt – it grew readily on the land fertilised by the Nile, and having a relatively reliable and abundant food source may have allowed Egyptian civilisation to become as advanced as it did. The grain supply was a political issue in ancient Rome – election campaigns often featured lowering the price of grain or offering free grain to the poor. Trade between the regions of the Roman empire increased the range of domesticated products available for consumption;

some species of food plants were subsequently adapted to new climates.

Contact between Europe and the Americas in the middle ages further altered the menu – the potato quickly became a successful crop, and in some areas replaced grains as the staple.

A step-change in the human relationship with grains occurred during the nineteenth century, when cheap polishing methods were discovered, allowing the creation of white flour on a large scale. Previously, refined products had only been available to a privileged few – now foods based on refined carbohydrates became cheap and easy to produce, and they were quickly established as staples for poorer people.

It was around the same time that breakfast cereals began to emerge in the US, initially popularised as health foods by the Rev. Sylvester Graham and then John Harvey Kellogg, both promoters of the moral benefits of a vegetarian diet. The turn of the century saw the large scale commercial production of highly profitable breakfast cereals, which soon became a national craze due to clever advertising. The addition of sugar to the products further increased their popularity, and entry to the global market came in the 1920s. Apart from during the Second World War, commercial cereals have been a feature on the majority of British breakfast tables ever since.

Breakfast cereals are now available in a variety of shapes and flavours, some claiming health benefits with their added vitamins and fibre. They remain highly profitable for manufacturers. Sweet cereals are marketed to children – their appeal heightened by free gifts and bright packaging, and the advertising messages around cereals are so pervasive that many adults consider certain varieties to be healthy choices – when even those products marketed as weight loss aids or being whole grain based are high in sugar or glucose-fructose syrup.

Grain-derived syrups themselves deserve a brief mention here. US subsidies of corn, and tariffs on imported cane sugar mean that syrups produced from corn are more cost effective as sweeteners, and have become difficult to avoid in convenience foods produced in America. Many British processed foods also contain them. Corn syrups all require modification by enzymes, and it is possible to control the proportions of different sugars within the syrup – high fructose corn syrup (HFCS) has a high fructose:glucose ratio and is therefore sweeter than cane or beet sugar. There are a number of arguments against the widespread use of HFCS and other corn syrups:

- Whilst derived from a natural source, it is not a sweetener that would exist in nature, and therefore has more detrimental effects on the body than fruit sugar, cane sugar or beet sugar
- Its low cost encourages over-consumption
- It adds calories to many products, not just those where a sweetener is expected – bread and savoury convenience foods often contain HFCS
- Some batches of HFCS manufactured in the US have been found to contain mercury, which is toxic
- The taste of products sweetened with HFCS as opposed to cane or beet sugar is inferior

Processed grains and their derivatives are generally best avoided but whole, unrefined grains can be part of a healthy diet. Studies have linked whole grain consumption with decreased risk of cardiovascular disease, diabetes and cancer, and it is not yet clear whether there is a specific component of whole grains that confers the benefit (for example, fibre, B vitamins, phytic acid). Some pieces of research have suggested that whole grain consumption is also correlated with a lower body fat percentage, and less abdominal fat storage.

The differences between individuals consuming whole grains and those who consume no grains at all are yet to be determined – generally, the amount of whole grains included in the diet should be determined on an individual basis – some people benefit from a grain-free or low-grain approach, whereas others thrive on diets where a significant proportion of calories are contributed by whole grains. Ability to digest grains is part of this – whilst true intolerance to gluten, a protein found in wheat, and to a lesser degree in some other grains, is rare, low level reactions such as bloating and altered bowel habit are common. Nutritional questionnaires, metabolic typing and BioSignature analysis may all be helpful in determining how well-suited a person is to carbohydrates; although trial and error and intelligent guesswork can be equally useful.

Care must be taken when choosing whole grain products, as the "whole grain" banner is used as a successful marketing tools. Many whole grain, 100% natural and organic products are still high in sugar, and should not be included regularly as part of a fat loss plan.

In conclusion, whilst the use of grain has accompanied the rise of human civilisations, it is possible that abuse of this convenient food source could damage the health of current and future generations. The power of the customer in a profit-driven food environment may provide a solution - through avoiding refined and processed grain products such as commercial breakfast cereals and HFCS, consumers can place their vote for a focus on grains that is beneficial for health, not merely for the profits of the food industry.

Chapter summary

- In September, get back into routines, and start modifying your lifestyle for the autumn
- Now might be a good time to begin taking supplements, if you don't already - certain supplements can help prevent colds, or can reduce their duration

- Think about the place of grain in your diet - it is a convenient food source, but it is abused by the modern food industry

Workbook section

Changes I have made this year to my diet and/or lifestyle:
e.g., Exercise type and frequency, lifestyle practices, foods I try to avoid

Changes that have been easy to make:

Changes that have been more difficult:

How I feel now, compared with earlier in the year:

What has worked best:

How I would like to continue, for next year, and the future:

What specifically I will plan to stop doing, either because it is unhelpful for my goals, or because it doesn't work for me or fit harmoniously into my life:

How I usually feel in autumn:

My thoughts about autumn:

Supplements I might try this season:

How I might modify my grain intake:

October

Winter is coming

October was the month when Northern European peoples such as the Anglo-Saxons recognised the coming of winter. In the Slavic languages that do not use the Latin month names, October is the yellow month (zhovten, Ukrainian), the time of falling leaves (listopad, Crotian), the month of broken flax stalks (Polish, Belarusian, padziernik, kastrichnik – relating to the harvest of flax), or the time where deer mate (říjen, Czech) – all related to the changes in nature. October includes the last harvests of fruit and grain.

During the Roman era, the feast of the goddess of Agriculture, Ceres, fell in October. Activities involved fasts, followed by games and feasting. In England, a church service for the Harvest of the Sea was held churches during October, and is still held today in some areas today, honouring the bounty of the sea. By far the best known event taking place during October is at the very end of the month – Halloween, or Samhain.

Halloween/Samhain is now mostly an opportunity for children and young people to make mischief and collect sweets, but it was an important occasion in Celtic countries. Whilst the belief that Samhain was the start of the Celtic New Year is most likely unfounded, tribal assemblies including discussions, feasting and games did take place in Mediaeval Ireland around the end of October/start of November.

As with the opening of the summer season in early May, the opening of the winter season in Celtic countries had a particular connection to the supernatural. The dead were honoured, the future was divined and it was considered prudent to guard against the activities of witches and spirits. In England, the time of the year was also associated with the supernatural, but there was a more fearful character to the English customs – families were especially concerned with warding off evil. The Christian feast of the dead, taking place on 1 November, was an important event throughout England, and it is the All Souls Day collections that may have given rise to modern trick or treat practices.

Samhain/Halloween was a minor festival in England until relatively recently, being focused perhaps on more regional and community-specific practices. It increased in popularity with Irish immigration, being popular in America due to the large Irish population. Pumpkins at Halloween, assumed to be an old part of the festival, are actually a relatively new introduction.

With night falling ever more rapidly and the weather turning colder, October is the month to begin a way of life more adapted to the darker months.

Time for reflection

Preparation for autumn should begin in September, as described in the previous chapter, since in addition to changes in seasonal energy, it is when many people return to routines after a more relaxed summer. September, though, has many of the characteristics of late summer – an "extra" season included in the Chinese perspective of the year.

Late summer is represented by the Earth element and the colour yellow. It has qualities of both stability and transformation, and as a period of harvest, it represents the result of the year's work. Despite these generally positive attributes, the emotions associated with the Earth element according to Chinese medicine are those of melancholy and worry; for agrarian people, anxiety around the success of the harvest was perhaps very real, and whilst summer involved hard work, it was also no doubt a time of easier living in some senses – and so autumn and winter, and the weather conditions they bring, would have been greeted with apprehension. Even where sustenance through the colder months is not an issue, the end of summer does have a particularly poignancy, with the end of holidays and carefree living, and the return to the grind.

Autumn, which is felt fully in October in England, is associated with the Metal element and ideas of letting go. Metal is usually buried in the earth – great abundance carries within it the beginnings of the next stage, that of loss, which is experienced in autumn. The emotion of autumn is grief, and its colour is white, the colour of death and bones - as this, not winter, is the season of paring down, and of endings. The cycle of the year is nearing completion, seeds nurtured through the last winter have sprouted, grown, matured and been harvested. Flowers and foliage are now falling away to reveal bare branches and fields, the foundations of the landscape. There are late harvests now, including apples and squashes, but after this, it would have been necessary to rely on the hardy winter crops and preserved food until spring.

The British climate is generally unpredictable, and in this vein autumn can bring frosts, as well as golden sunny days. Trees shed their leaves at different times, and so some varieties appear to be holding on to summer, whilst others have given in to the cold winds already. It can therefore be difficult to set a pace – in September, whilst starting to think about the change of season, many people take on new activities, resume those discontinued during summer, or retain more expansive summer habits. Now, begin to hold back energy as the time for storage approaches. This could mean setting aside more quiet time, and reflecting on the past year and your priorities.

Christmas products are available from October in many shops, which serves as a reminder that the winter solstice is approaching.

Getting into an autumn rhythm

Winter often requires practical adaptations – the weather is cold, and so warming foods may be particularly useful and appealing;

in terms of exercise, outdoor activities may need to be limited or modified. Such changes may not feel necessary in early autumn, although making more subtle alterations to your lifestyle in line with the season may help to protect energy levels and general wellbeing. Some ideas are given here:

- If you find the darkening mornings difficult, where possible, allow yourself a little longer in bed whilst continuing to avoid large variations in your waking and sleeping times
- Wiccans use rituals to welcome the seasons – perhaps arrange a practical "ritual" of your own, to mark the change:
    - Make a point of putting away summer clothes and shoes, and perhaps invest in some new autumn/winter pieces
    - Think about adding warmer colours to your home environment, perhaps creating a flower arrangement involving autumn leaves, or using throws and cushions
- Whenever possible, take time over preparing and eating meals. Eating seasonally and locally can be relatively easy, even when shopping at supermarkets
- To make the most of summer, it is common to rush from activity to activity. Now, consciously slow down
- Before evaluating an exercise programme from a practical perspective, consider it more intuitively – autumn may feel suited to more strength and flexibility work, as opposed to cardiovascular fitness. Conversely, outdoor activity in the cooler weather may be invigorating for some

The importance of light: SAD and winter blues

In our 24-hour society, little attention is given to natural light levels, but for most of history, they would have dictated the activities of the day, as well as of the time of year. Once darkness fell, little outdoor work would have been possible, and candles would have afforded the only way to continue with indoor work such as weaving or sewing.

Many animals demonstrate changes in behaviour throughout the year, with a significant proportion of species hibernating during the winter months. The same is true of plants, which go to seed, or shed their leaves in autumn. It could be argued that the lower mood and lethargy exhibited by some humans during autumn and winter is a natural adaptation, that is simply out of kilter with the modern way of life.

The term Seasonal Affective Disorder (SAD) covers all season-related changes in mental health, although most commonly it refers to depressive symptoms in autumn/winter, which improve in spring. Clinically, it is not considered to be separate from major depression, but as an association of it. Recurrence every year for at least 2 years, with remission in the spring, is required for diagnosis. There may be a connection between unipolar depression, SAD and bipolar affective disorder.

Typical features of autumn/winter SAD include:

- Difficulty getting up in the morning, low morning energy,
- Disturbed sleep, and/or a tendency to oversleep
- Generally low energy and reduced libido
- Carbohydrate cravings
- Low mood
- Feeling of being unable to cope, anxiety
- "Fuzzy" thinking

Remission in the spring may be preceded by a period of manic activity or anxiety, or may be gradual. There is also a pattern of SAD whereby symptoms of anxiety and mania dominate, occurring during spring and summer. Some sufferers experience both lethargy and low mood in autumn/winter, and hypomania during spring and summer – demonstrating the connection with bipolar affective disorder.

SAD is not to be confused with the state of simply not enjoying autumn and winter weather, feeling less inclined to be outdoors because of wind and rain, or turning towards more restful activities on dark, chilly evenings. SAD can have a large impact on a person's life. A sociable and motivated individual may become withdrawn and anxious, unable to complete their usual tasks or concentrate on work. A milder form of seasonal mood/behaviour change is known as winter blues, where sufferers feel more lethargic during autumn and winter, but do not have functioning impaired to such an extent.

There are likely to be a number of subtypes of SAD and winter blues, with a variety of causes, although underexposure to natural light is a key causative factor in all cases. Light regulates the balance of neurotransmitters, such as serotonin, the "happy" hormone, and melatonin, the hormone of sleep. Low levels of light correspond with low levels of serotonin, and higher levels of melatonin, resulting in lower mood and increased sleepiness – light is the switch for the body to stop producing melatonin, which is why waking up earlier in summer tends to be easier. Research has shown the effect of light on serotonin as well as the positive effects of light therapy in SAD.

The picture is unlikely to be as simple as a serotonin/melatonin imbalance alone – individual circadian rhythms, lifestyle and genetic predisposition may also be involved. Other medical problems and functional imbalances can also exacerbate SAD or winter blues symptoms.

Do you have SAD/winter blues?

Consider the following carefully, and think about whether you might benefit from SAD/winter blues treatment. Speak with your

GP if you think you might be suffering from depression.

Q: Do you find it more difficult to get out of bed during autumn and winter?

Humans wake naturally with light, and in the depths of winter it may not become light until time to leave for work, so it is unsurprising that dark mornings are difficult. Few people relish the prospect of getting up in the dark, but there is a difference between wanting to spend an extra half hour in bed, and finding getting up an almost superhuman challenge.

If the latter describes you well, consider a dawn simulator to wake you with light – even though the dawn may still be a few hours away. If you also have symptoms of general low energy, consider a SAD lamp to use throughout the day.

Q: Do you usually put on weight (fat) throughout the darker, colder months?

Weight (fat) gain in autumn and winter is common, due to decreased activity levels, carbohydrate cravings, (and the ever-presence of the foods to satisfy these cravings), and may even have once been a useful adaptation, to make the most of scarce winter foods.

Consider using a SAD lamp, and/or 5-HTP (see February chapter) to boost serotonin levels, which may reduce carbohydrate cravings. Also make sure you are providing your body with the food it needs – adding carbohydrate treats in occasionally is then less of a problem.

Finally, if you are gaining fat and your will power is particularly low, avoid buying starchy carbohydrates. At other times, it may be possible to have biscuits and cakes in the house for treats, and to be able to ignore their presence for most of the time. This is less likely during the darker months, so where possible, decrease you exposure to refined carbohydrates, sweet, junk food and any other "triggers".

Q: Do you feel lower in mood and more lethargic in autumn and winter?

There is much at this time of year that can be considered draining, but if you find you are particularly affected by the change of season, finding life significantly more difficult (rather than feeling let down by the weather, or more inclined to stay at home in the darker evenings), SAD or winter blues interventions may help. If you are increasingly unable to cope, and the symptoms are affecting your life, see your doctor.

Treating SAD

There is evidence that bright light therapy is helpful for sufferers of SAD and winter blues – and indeed it may be helpful for non-seasonal chronic depression. Light boxes and SAD lamps are made to certain specifications – they must provide light at a certain intensity in order to be effective. Depending on the model, 15-60 minutes of exposure per day are required, so choose carefully – a light, portable model may be best for you, or an attractively styled model that could be an elegant part of the design of your home or office. See the Resources section for more information on manufacturers and websites.

Natural light therapies (such as Real Sunlight), involving all frequencies of light – visible, infra red and UV are now available. The UV rays are at a lesser intensity than found in natural sunlight, and therefore do not damage the skin. Such products do not easily cause tanning.

Negative ion therapy has also been shown to relieve SAD, winter blues and improve chronic depressive symptoms. Negative ions are molecules or atoms with an extra electron, giving them an overall negative charge. They cause positively charged or neutral pollutant molecules to stick together, becoming heavier and falling under gravity, rather than being suspended in the air. Their effect on mood is somewhat mysterious, but has been documented. Negative ion generators are easily available and can be relatively inexpensive.

Antidepressant medication can be helpful for SAD, but speak to your GP and consider the options carefully.

Finally, it is particularly important for SAD/winter blues sufferers to ensure other aspects of their diet and lifestyle are optimised. Regular exercise will help to boost both energy levels and mood, and will help to establish healthy sleep patterns. Satisfying carbohydrate cravings with good quality, natural and unprocessed carbohydrates, and the occasional good-quality treat, instead of regularly indulging in sweets and refined carbohydrate products, will help to prevent weight (fat) gain, as well as supporting energy levels.

The importance of light: Vitamin D

As well as regulating mood and affecting cognition, light is required for the production of vitamin D.

UVB rays act on 7-dehydroxycholesterol in the skin, converting it to 25-OH vitamin D. This is then activated in the kidneys to form the hormonally active calcitriol (1,25-OH vitamin D). Vitamin D is fat soluble, and can be stored in the body – reserves built up during summer can be used throughout the rest of the year.

The importance of vitamin D for preventing rickets (in children) and weak bones (in adults) is well known, and for decades it was assumed that this was its only role. Intake did not have to be large to prevent the disease – as well as being formed in the skin, vitamin D can be obtained from fish and fortified dairy products, and exposure to the sun need only be minimal to obtain the required amount.

Recently, though, it was discovered that receptors for

calcitriol are found on a wide variety of body cells, suggesting its effects are far reaching.

Vitamin D deficiency is thought to affect the following areas:

- Bone health
- Immune system balance
- Risk of colorectal, breast and prostate cancer
- Cardiovascular risk
- Allergic diseases such as asthma and eczema
- Skin problems such as psoriasis

Maintaining healthy vitamin D levels during pregnancy and breast feeding is particularly important, as prenatal and/or early life deficiency may be implicated in multiple sclerosis (which is more prevalent in countries with lower levels of light – Scotland has a high MS rate due to its latitude and cloud cover levels) and mental health problems including schizophrenia.

Deficiency is a particular problem in the UK as there are many barriers to the population obtaining sufficient vitamin D from the sun, and the typical British diet is not rich in the substance. Fish was once a staple in Scotland, supplying adequate vitamin D, but this is no longer the case.

For at least six out of twelve months, optimal vitamin D production in the skin is not possible in Britain as the sun is too low in the sky – the UV rays that cause the formation of vitamin D are filtered out by the atmosphere. In summer, when vitamin D reserves should be built up, there is frequently too much cloud cover for adequate penetration of UV rays. When conditions for vitamin D production do exist (right time of year, little cloud cover), it would be necessary to regularly expose the arms and shoulders to the sun at midday, without sunscreen, for at least 15 minutes – and few people are able to do this.

In the past, vitamin D deficiency may have been less of a problem as in addition to a diet richer in the vitamin, life was less indoor-focused. Even those with jobs indoors would have spent more time outdoors travelling, relaxing and carrying out tasks such as shopping. Importantly, children now spend significantly less time outdoors than even a generation ago. Supplementation may therefore be required for many people in Britain.

How do I know how much vitamin D3 I need?

Severe vitamin D deficiency in adults may cause weak bones, but sub-optimal levels may not be detectable without a test, and could have longer term implications for health. If you are Asian or black, you are at greater risk of vitamin D deficiency (vitamin D is made less efficiently in darker skin); overweight people are also more likely to be vitamin D deficient. Request a vitamin D blood test from your GP, or from a private laboratory to provide you with a better understanding of your vitamin D status.

The current RDA for vitamin D of 400IU may be too low – it is sufficient to prevent rickets, but not enough to correct a longstanding deficiency, or to optimise levels in people who do not receive large amounts of vitamin D from their diets, or from outdoor living. Some researchers recommend much higher doses of vitamin D, working from the fact that exposure to sunlight can generate 10,000IU of vitamin D in less than an hour. Depending on your test results, you may need to exceed the RDA to achieve optimal levels.

There are fears, which are largely unfounded, around increasing the RDA of vitamin D. It is thought that high vitamin D intakes could cause blood calcium levels to rise to dangerously high levels, although this is unlikely to happen, unless another illness, or calcium system abnormality is already present. Those with sarcoid or other causes of hypercalcaemia, or TB, should not use vitamin D supplements, and if using high dosages of vitamin D, it is advisable to have regular blood tests to ensure levels remain within normal limits – the substance is stored in the body, and so it is possible to exceed normal levels relatively quickly.

When choosing a vitamin D supplement, choose vitamin D3 as this is more easily absorbed than D2. Read the directions carefully, particularly where liquid supplements are concerned – some products offer 1000IU per drop.

Chapter summary

- Reflect on the qualities of autumn this month, and make intuitive changes to your exercise programme
- If you think you have symptoms of SAD or winter blues, speak to your doctor and also look into the natural approaches to dealing with this. A SAD lamp or light box can be very helpful for reducing symptoms
- Have your vitamin D levels tested and consider supplementation - deficiency and sub-optimal levels are both very common in the UK and can have a variety of consequences for health

Workbook section

How I usually feel at this time of year:

What I will do this year in order to feel better:

Ways in which I will start to turn my energies inwards:

Signs of approaching winter I have noticed:

Winter

Nurture
Re-charge
Energy focused inwards

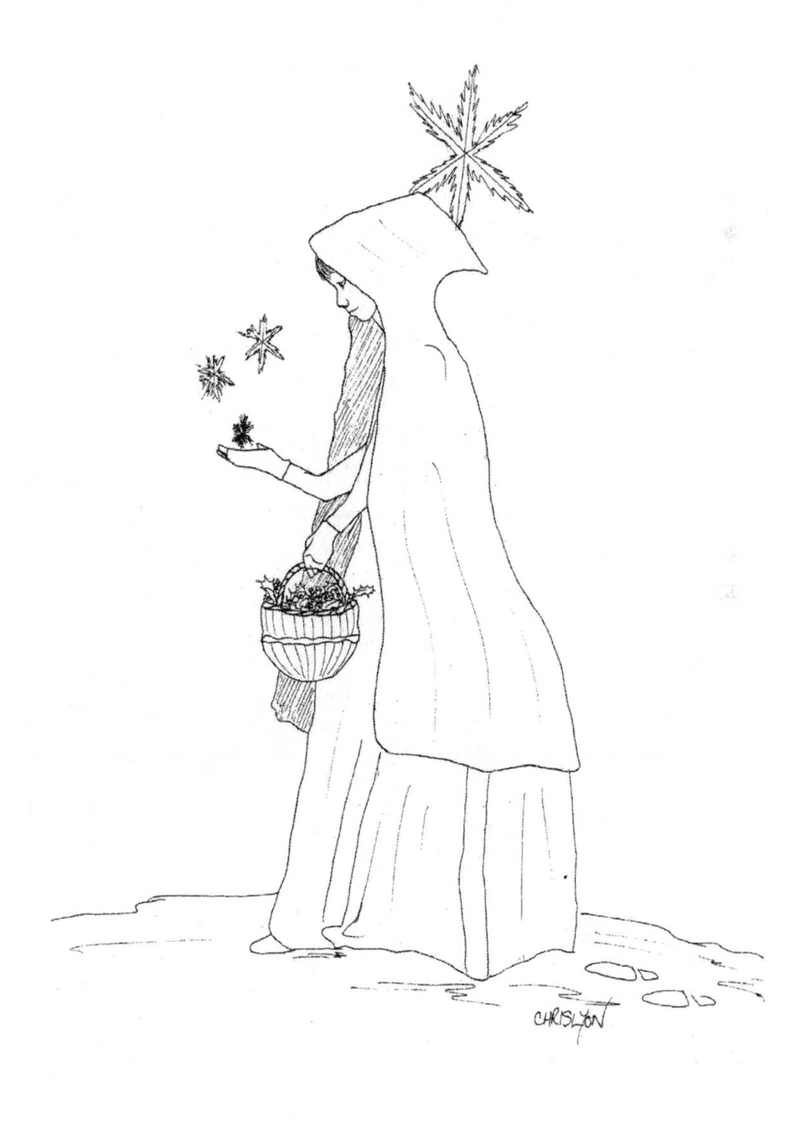

November

The dark part of the year

There are many associations between death and the month of November. In the majority of Slavic languages, it is known as listopad, leaf-fall, as it is a time when leaves die and trees become bare. The Christian feasts of All Saints and All Souls, which honour the dead, fall on 1 and 2 November respectively, and the day for remembering those killed in wars, Remembrance Day, falls on 11 November.

The Anglo-Saxons called November Blood month, as it was the month when the cattle that were not to be kept during the winter were slaughtered. It was the last opportunity to have fresh meat until spring. Slaughtering at the start of winter remained a yearly practice, and it usually took place by 11 November, St Martin's Day. This was probably an occasion for fun and indulgence, in the face of the rapidly increasing darkness.

St Martin's day may have been the last opportunity for celebration until Christmas for many English citizens, although the date of the accession of Queen Elizabeth (17 November) was celebrated in some towns and cities, and in certain areas the feast of St Nicholas in early December was also marked. St Nicholas' Day celebrations are still popular in some European countries.

The fifth of November became a day of national celebration after Guy Fawkes' foiled attempt at treason in 1605 – it was an occasion for giving thanks for the preservation of the government, although its popularity may be explained by it providing an opportunity for distraction from the harshness of the season. It was during the Victorian era that bonfires became public events, bringing together communities, rather than being held in more private spaces. The night of 5 November was seen as an opportunity for mischief, and today it is still enjoyed for its light-hearted aspects – fireworks, the bonfire and toffee apples.

Thanksgiving is celebration on the 4th Thursday in November in the US. It is an occasion to give thanks for the harvest, and has been celebrated for several centuries, since the European settlers survived through the preceding harsh winter.

November should be a time to resist the feelings of darkness and drabness, and to enjoy a nurturing winter season.

What does winter mean for you?

Do you see winter as a magical time for connection with others, a time for reflection and being alone, or a dreary season of cold and darkness? The following questions will help clarify your attitude towards winter.

Which of the following best describes how you view winter overall?

a) Winter is a time to get cosy and spend time with family and friends
b) Winter is a time to spend time by myself, working on my own projects
c) Winter is a time I dread, which I just need to "get through"

Winter living

a) I like winter clothing styles, and look forward to shopping for a new winter wardrobe
b) I like the colder temperatures at this time of year, and how natural scenes are often starkly beautiful. I enjoy the slower pace of life
c) I dislike having to wrap up warm, prepare for bad weather, etc

Winter eating

a) I enjoy experimenting with different flavours, textures

and spices in winter

b) In winter, I enjoy simple, filling foods, such as the naturally available root vegetables
c) I don't enjoy the stodgy foods typically eaten in winter

Winter exercise

a) I tend to continue to exercise during winter, I enjoy winter sports and so need to stay in shape for the season
b) I tend to slow down in winter in terms of exercise, but do enjoy brisk walks in the countryside
c) I find it difficult to motivate myself to exercise in winter, because of the darkness and cold weather

What your answers mean

Mostly A

You are likely to be someone who enjoys the family gatherings and feasts of winter, and do not tend to feel drained by the season. You don't find cold weather off-putting, and may enjoy winter sports – so staying in shape throughout is not difficult. You see winter as an opportunity to experiment with a wider range of food textures, flavours and spices, and enjoy creating and sharing warming stews and soups.

Mostly B

You appreciate the quieter nature of the season, the sense of drawing in. You see it as a period for focusing on the essentials, and for spending time alone. You enjoy the simplicity of a pared-down version of nature – bare branches, especially when glistening with frost, do not seem dead to you, but clean and starkly beautiful. Whilst you often slow down during winter, you continue to be active, perhaps taking long walks in the countryside. After the experiments of spring and summer and the abundance of autumn, winter food represents simplicity for you warming, uncomplicated dishes, often based on what is seasonally available.

Mostly C
Winter is far from your favourite season, you tend to find it difficult – the darkness may affect you, causing SAD or winter blues (see October), and the cold weather further discourages you from being active. You prefer the lighter living of summer.

Now thinking about your answers, and using information on light from the previous chapter, and on the immune system from the September chapter, take the space at the end of this chapter to record your own action plan. If you find winter difficult, the following section about reframing may be particularly useful.

Reframing the time of year

Maintaining health, fitness and wellbeing initiatives throughout the whole year should not be problematic, indeed those keen on winter sports may find activity levels increase during winter, and the need for heartier dishes can make cooking more interesting at this time.

Winter is often viewed negatively, however, and it is not difficult to see why – at first glance, nature appears to have shut down. Foliage has mostly withered, animals hibernate and humans take comfort where they can. Summer encourages expansiveness, but now we are drawn to take shelter, to hurry home after a hard day where daylight may have been barely seen, to skip extra activities such as exercise, and to reach for easily prepared, satisfying foods.

Winter is a time of preparation, though, and should be viewed as such. Many edible plants come into season in winter, as starchy roots are the plant's energy store for the colder months. Rather than turning energy outwards, in the production of leaves and flowers, the plant directs energy underground, into storing and protecting. Winter is an important period horticulturally, for cutting back on old growth to make way for spring.

As blossoms would not be seen in spring without quiet, determined work throughout the winter, in terms of making progress with improving wellbeing, or losing fat, this is an opportunity for focus. Schedules may need to be pared down, more time spent resting and meals adapted to provide warmth and sustain energy, but this is not a time of stasis or regression. Pick out the most important aspects of your plan, and ensure these are not lost. Not only will continued commitment to healthier living lead to rewards that can be enjoyed during the warmer months, but it will improve the experience of winter itself.

Avoiding winter fat gain

Food

Food should be enjoyed, and is not merely a physical experience. However, it is possible to become caught in a negative cycle of dependence of foods, or certain patterns of consumption, particularly at this time of year. Identify the foods and drinks you tend to reach for to provide comfort – this could be chocolate, wine or crisps, and commit to doing without them for 5 days of the week at least. This will help to break down the associations between the food and the emotions.

Be honest about how winter affects you – carbohydrate cravings and low will power may mean that starchy carbohydrates should not be in the cupboard, and that treats should be enjoyed away from home. Do not allow "slips" to degenerate into a downwards spiral, and realise when you might be more vulnerable than usual to making unhealthy food choices (e.g.,pre-menstrually, during periods of work stress).

Also look at specific situations where will power disappears, which might be social gatherings, or when at home watching a film, and make an effort to be disciplined the next time this takes place. Once you have enjoyed one film without the usual pizza or ice cream, or socialised without being drunk, your habits have already started to change and you are on the way to being back in control. A friend or partner might be able to help you make the first step here.

It is also worth considering how other aspects of your lifestyle could be changed – winter has its difficulties, but planning new activities or reviewing your routines can help to keep you away from unhelpful patterns.

During this period, include protein with every meal, to help keep blood sugar levels balanced, and make an extra effort to plan meals in advance. Keeping the freezer stocked with portions of home-made casserole, and a pot of soup in the fridge, means you have easy access to tasty, healthy meals, when the idea of cooking from scratch becomes unappealing. You might not enjoy snacking on cold foods now, so try roasted vegetables sprinkled with seeds, small portions of soup or boiled eggs instead. Herbal teas are warming and can satisfy the craving to "consume something" – experiment with different flavours.

Exercise

If you respond well to having an exercise routine and clear goals, and if you are already in the habit of exercising, you should not find keeping active during winter a challenge, as you will simply stick to your plans, whatever the weather. If you are yet to begin exercise, the key is to overcome any initial inertia, perhaps by working out with friends, or booking a Personal Training session – then commitment to a plan for the rest of the winter is quite likely. Setting goals to reach by the end of the year could be another motivating factor.

Individuals who exercise out of compulsion, or who have an all or nothing approach to diet and lifestyle, should seek balance during the colder months. Avoiding peaks and troughs in blood sugar, through choosing foods sensibly, can be helpful in reducing feelings of instability, and regular exercise can relieve tension and generate "feel-good" neurotransmitters. If an "all or nothing" approach has meant that exercise has fallen by the wayside in winter, start getting back on track with small changes. Walk, rather than take public transport, and then try out a fun-sounding activity to warm up. Ask a friend to accompany you to the gym, have a brisk walk in the country one weekend and perhaps spend a day in some conservation volunteering – before you know it, you will have had several exercise sessions and can congratulate yourself on being back on plan! The next stage would be to come back to training and making progress each time you work out.

For those who require intellectual stimulation to be part of a work out, or who are easily bored, continuing to exercise can be a challenge when energy reserves are decreased – you most likely want to direct them towards other areas. An answer may be found in planning short but intense exercise sessions, allowing physical activity to be "got out of the way". Once fitness improves, activity may become more appealing for its own sake.

If exercising outdoors during autumn and winter, remember that equipment may need to be changed.

Warm up!

The first days requiring gloves and scarves are usually in late October or early November, as frosts and icy winds become more common, so it is useful to look at warming up from a number of perspectives.

Activity raises body temperature, and so intersperse sedentary work with movement, and when exercising, be sure to go through a warm up routine. This is important at any time of the year, but is of particular concern when the body temperature may be initially low, or when exercise sessions take place in a colder space.

Consider borrowing customs from countries with colder winters – ice skating, sauna bathing and sharing spiced teas and wines with others can all help to brighten up dull, chilly days.

Warming up with food

Winter food should be satisfying and warming – richer game meats, root vegetables and spices are all welcome now. From the Chinese medical perspective, there are a number of ways to classify food:

- Temperature energy - hot, warm, neutral, cool or cold
- Taste - sweet, salty, sour, bitter, spicy
- Fullness, which relates to the food's ability to build, or to help elimination
- Dampening or drying effect

Some of these properties fit easily with Western ideas, yet others can be a little surprising – for example, beef is a warm, sweet, full food. Some spices, whilst having a hot energy, can be empty in quality – meaning they are useful for elimination, and can actually cool and purify the body.

Some hot and warming foods include:

- Lamb
- Chicken
- Anchovy
- Turkey
- Goat's cheese
- Onion
- Garlic
- Winter squash
- Kale
- Walnut
- Pine nut

- Date
- Coffee
- Black tea
- Chocolate

The following are some insights from the energetic method of eating:

- Cow's milk dairy products are neutral in energy, and so should be reduced when the weather is cold – adding cinnamon to yogurt is a way to increase its warmth
- Green tea is considered to be cooling, so in winter, perhaps blend it with ginger
- Salad ingredients such as cucumber, lettuce, tomato and celery are all cold or cool, and from a Chinese perspective should be minimised in winter, as should fruits such as bananas, melons, strawberries and oranges
- Any fruits eaten during winter should be cooked and served with spices
- Excessive hot or cold energy foods should be avoided. A particular cold energy food to be wary of is sugar
- In a damp climate such as the UK, avoiding dampening foods such as flour products, raw foods, dairy products, excessive fruit and soy products may be helpful for some people.

Thinking of skiing this winter?

Skiing and snowboarding are some of the most popular outdoor activities for winter, even though they are not part of the culture for most of the UK. They provide great workouts, particularly for the lower body, and cross country skiing is excellent for improving endurance.

If you are thinking of a skiing or snowboarding holiday this winter, consider the careful preparation that should be done in advance to make sure you are in top shape and less likely to be injured – even if you are a veteran. Squats and lunges are important lower body exercises that will strengthen the muscles and joints used in skiing and snowboarding. Supplements such as glucosamine and chondroitin are widely used for joint health, and many people find them useful, although there is little scientific evidence for their effectiveness.

Double check equipment to make sure it is all still safe to use, and adequate for your needs. If you haven't been on the slopes for some time, consider booking a refresher lesson.

Preparing for the festive season

The festive season can provide joyful opportunities to reconnect with friends and family, and enjoy celebrations during the darkest, coldest months. It can also be a time of stress, and where healthy lifestyle initiatives are compromised. The December chapter deals with the festive season in detail, but spend some time in November planning the festivities.

A common problem during the festive season is trying to please everyone, which is extremely draining. Focus on the essentials, which are more likely to

include opportunities to spend quality time with others, as opposed to specifications for the Christmas spread. If buying presents becomes a financial strain, consider agreeing with certain family members not to buy, or set a price limit, and if parties and gatherings become a chore, limit them.

Chapter summary

- Now many people find it hard to resist the temptation of desserts and excessive starchy carbohydrates. Identify your triggers and be honest with yourself – this may be the time to avoid having these foods in the house. You may also need to expend more effort in planning meals now – if healthy, warming food is available, you are less likely to make choices that lead to lethargy or fat gain

- If you find winter difficult, remind yourself that it is a period of preparation - energy is turned inwards, and spring blossoms would not be possible without the quiet work of plants throughout the colder months
- Exercising during winter may require a different approach. If planning a skiing holiday, make sure you are in good shape and have attended to musculoskeletal problems

Workbook section

Reflections on the time of year – changes noticed in nature recently and in how I feel:

Action plan for the colder, darker months

How I usually feel in autumn/winter:

What I want to be different this year:

How I will support my immune system:

How I will combat the lack of light, if this affects me:

How I will stay active:

How I will ensure I eat tastily, but healthily:

Ideas for brightening up the time of year:

What I am looking forward to this season:

How I might need to change aspects of my lifestyle:
(e.g., may prefer to stop exercising outdoors, add different supplements, swap some water intake for tea)

December

Festive joy

The last month of the year brings parties, family gatherings and national days of celebration. Christmas has been celebrated in England for over a millennium, although its historical link with the birth of Jesus Christ is tenuous. The choice of the timing of the celebration may have been more influenced by pagan celebrations of the winter solstice and the beginning of the return of the sun, which the early church saw were popular, than by any historical events.

The pagan solstice festivals in ancient Rome are likely to have their origins in an older Syrian cult. The darkest time of the year has a focus on light, as once the winter solstice has passed, the days gradually begin to lengthen.

Prior to the adoption of the Syrian cult, there were important Roman festivals before and after the solstice – Saturnalia took place in the days after 17 December, and the New Year feast of the Kalendae on 1 to 3 January. Saturnalia, in honour of Saturn, involved several days of public holiday, gambling, games and feasting. Presents were often given, particularly candles. The Kalendae, dedicated to Janus, involved the exchange of gifts to bring luck in the coming year.

It is not clear whether or how the winter solstice was celebrated in pre-Christian Britain, but it was believed to be important for Norse peoples, and the Anglo-Saxons were thought to have celebrated "Mother Night" at or near to the solstice.

During the middle ages, more and more days around the Christmas period were given over to celebrations, culminating in the establishment of the 12 days of Christmas, including a number of saints' days and the New Year celebrations and ending with the major feast of the Epiphany on 6 January.

Today Christmas parties begin early in December, if not late November, but the weeks before Christmas – Advent – were previously given over to fasting and abstinence. Feasting began on Christmas day, when local lords would provide feasts for the villagers.

Gifts were initially part of the New Year, rather than the Christmas celebrations - although this practice died out by the early 19th century. Giving gifts of money to apprentices, servants and tradesmen became habitual during the 17th and 18th centuries, and charity at this time continues with the name Boxing Day (from Christmas boxes). Fancy dress (mumming) and particular drinking rituals (wassailing) were popular throughout the middle ages around Christmastime.

From 1610 onwards, specific foods such as mince pies, plum pudding and hot spiced ale with apples were all part of Christmas. Many of the Christmas traditions remained in England even after the reformation, although this was not the case in Scotland.

Celebrations around the winter solstice have most likely been taking place for over two thousand years, and for almost a thousand, Christmas has been an important time of year. Certain practices recognised today are centuries old, but it was in the Victorian era that many of the aspects of Christmas that we recognise today came into being – it lost the character of a series of public celebrations, and became family focused.

The festive season can be an opportunity to resist the darkness of midwinter by enjoying time with family and friends, and feasting. Whilst restorative holidays are experienced by many people, the modern interpretation of this period is generally based on stress, overeating, overdrinking and overspending. It can therefore be fraught with difficulty for people trying to live healthily, and is usually a prelude to resolutions and frugality in the early part of the New Year.

Food and the festive season

Food plays a large part in winter celebrations, and Christmas is generally connected with overindulgence. In England, it is common for families to stockpile biscuits, cakes and wine, as well as enjoying turkey, mince pies and Christmas pudding. Throughout this feasting, 1 January looms as the start of a grim period of payback, and the "all or nothing" mentality this represents can make longer term wellbeing and fat loss initiatives more difficult.

Do you have all or nothing behaviour?

If you answer yes to any of the following, you may have some typical "all or nothing" behaviours and should address these to maintain health and wellbeing and a consistent weight/body fat percentage. The more statements you feel that apply to you, the more you may need to work at finding balance.

- When I start a new fitness programme or diet, I can take it to extremes
- My emotional state can have a large impact on whether I eat healthily or not
- I sometimes binge
- When I overeat, I try to make up for it by not eating the next day, or eating very little
- Food is strongly associated with reward and punishment for me
- I think of some, if not most, foods as "bad"
- My weight tends to vary widely – at some point my wardrobe may have included size 8 clothes, and at others, size 16

Eating healthily, without self-deprivation

Being aware of food is one of the most important aspects of enjoying the festivities without overeating. It should be applied beyond this time of year, but December is a good month to begin, as there are ample opportunities for practice.

Obtaining and preparing food would have been a major focus of human life for millennia, requiring skill, thought and the expenditure of physical energy. Nowadays, thought must be exercised in order to avoid excess calorie intake – unnatural, energy dense foods are ubiquitous, being offered on the high street, in shops and supermarkets, in the workplace, at stations, on trains and even in hospitals and gyms. These carefully designed products are appealing, convenient and profitable for their manufacturers, but other than being a source of immediate energy, they tend to offer little in the way of nutrition. Additives required to improve shelf life, colour, texture or flavour have poorly understood effects on the body, and may be harmful (see the discussion of grains in the September chapter), and the environmental impact of manufacturing food products must also be taken into account. In this time of plenty, it is necessary to be selective about the types of food eaten.

Most of what a person eats should be food to sustain and nourish the body – food that is needed. These sorts of foods would include good quality protein, natural fats, vegetables and some whole grains. Food can also be eaten simply because it is enjoyable, and a wellbeing or fat loss plan should also allow for the inclusion of favourite foods and treats.

The final category comprises foods that are eaten out of habit, coercion or simply because they are available – this sort of eating should be minimised as much as possible, but is common during the festive season.

Becoming more aware of food

List foods under the categories given below (some examples are shown). Clarifying how you relate to different foods may be helpful for festive season eating.

Foods/drinks that are part of my fat loss/wellbeing plan, and that I enjoy:

e.g., grass fed beef steak

Foods/drinks that are part of my fat loss/wellbeing plan that I don't particularly enjoy, but should make more of an effort to eat:

e.g., fish, salads

Foods/drinks that are not part of my fat loss/wellbeing plan that I enjoy a lot:

e.g., home-made cakes

Foods/drinks that are not part of my fat loss/wellbeing plan, that I do not particularly enjoy, but which I end up eating quite often:

e.g., sandwiches

Foods/drinks I try to avoid:

e.g., dairy products (because of lactose intolerance)

Eating the foods in the first group is easy, because they are enjoyable. Some effort has to be made to include the foods in the second group – look up recipes that might make them more interesting; combine them with a home made sauce, or team with a more well liked meal element. The third groups represents foods that should be allowed as occasional treats.

The fourth group includes foods that you should plan to avoid – in the example given, sandwiches are an unhelpful food and not a source of enjoyment, most likely eaten because of convenience. Planning lunches and snacks may eliminate or greatly reduce the need for foods such as these. In some cases it may not be possible to remove these foods entirely, but making a healthier choice is always possible – plan oats instead of a refined and sweetened cereal, a hand-made sandwich on rye bread instead of a packaged version.

Some foods seem to fall between the third and fourth category, cheap, easily available foods often eaten on the go that do taste nice – commercial biscuits, chocolate bars, crisps and flapjacks, for example. Cutting down on these requires practice of delayed gratification, foregoing the "semi-treat" and looking forward to truly delicious food, once or twice a week.

The last column covers foods that should be avoided, perhaps because they cause feelings of bloatedness, or because they have an "addictive" potential. It can be difficult to avoid some of these during the festive season, where there is pressure from others to "have a good time".

Digestive Rescue

Even if you can be mindful throughout the festive season, different styles of cooking and richer dishes can often mean digestive upsets.

IBS

Irritable bowel syndrome (IBS) is a common condition – its cause is unknown, and there may indeed be a range of causes and triggers, ranging from hypersensitivity due to a poor nerve supply to the bowel, stress, sensitivity to certain foods, intestinal infections and irregular eating habits. It is a "functional" disorder, where there is no structural abnormality in the bowel.

Symptoms include excessive gas, bloating and the attendant discomfort, painful bowel spasms and diarrhoea and/or constipation.

Medical management may involve a range of investigations, to rule out other disorders, such as inflammatory bowel disease (IBD – a very different disease). Once IBS seems to be the most likely cause, there are only a few options – peppermint oil, or an antispasmodic, such as mebeverine. These can control the symptoms, although getting to the root of the problem may be more helpful. The sections below relate to IBS and isolated digestive upsets. See your doctor if your bowel habit has changed, and/or if you have noticed blood in your stools.

Identifying the culprits

Wheat and other gluten-containing grains, dairy products and foods containing yeast are all common culprits for both occasional digestive disturbances and IBS attacks.

Gluten, a protein found in grains, can cause severe problems in susceptible individuals, but this situation (coeliac disease) is relatively rare. Smaller scale sensitivity to gluten or other grain components is common, and manifests with discomfort and bloating after eating large amounts of grain-based foods. The only real strategy for improvement is avoidance. After a grain-free period, it may be possible to introduce occasional meals including grains with no ill effects.

Digestive symptoms following dairy consumption are usually due to a degree of lactose intolerance – this is not an allergy or sensitivity, but an enzyme deficiency (see March chapter).

Much is made in some alternative therapy circles about the importance of yeast – it is claimed that many health problems can be traced to overgrowth of yeast in the gut, particularly when this is coupled with a "leaky gut". Yeasts are a subtype of fungi, and make up part of the normal gut and skin flora in humans. The best known type of yeast in terms of health is *Candida albicans*, which causes vaginal and oral thrush when its growth becomes excessive.

Leaky gut involves an increase in the permeability of the gut wall, allowing bacteria, their toxins and food antigens to enter the blood stream. It is claimed that leaky gut is involved in conditions as diverse as autism, chronic fatigue syndrome, eczema and schizophrenia, and its symptoms can range from abdominal pain to hair loss and recurrent infections. It can be caused by infections, candida overgrowth and poor diet and lifestyle. Studies have confirmed that there may be increased intestinal permeability in patients with chronic fatigue syndrome, and it is possible that further connections will, in time be supported by research – although for now, leaky gut remains relatively mysterious.

Similarly, whilst candida is purported to underlie many kinds of ill health, most candida overgrowth studies relate to the familiar scenarios of oral and vaginal candidiasis, or to candida overgrowth occurring in the very ill, or immunosuppressed patient. Concerning the links between candida and wider health problems, there is some evidence for recurrent vaginal candidiasis being related to impaired glucose tolerance.

Whilst studies are yet to fully support the notion that candida and/or leaky gut are important contributors to a range of disease states, experiencing digestive symptoms after consuming yeast-containing products, such as beer, wine, vinegar and bread, is not uncommon, and some people also find that yeast or fungal conditions (such as athlete's foot) worsen when such products are included in the diet regularly. Whether or not this is due to existing yeast overgrowth in the gut is not certain, but yeast-containing foods are another category to potentially be wary of if you suffer from regular digestive disturbances or bloating, or if you have existing fungal infections, including thrush.

Overall, one of the most effective weapons against common functional digestive problems is keeping a diary. Whilst wheat, dairy and yeasts are commonly involved in causing bloating, discomfort, diarrhoea or constipation, recording when digestive disturbances occur in relation to food and stress may help you uncover a pattern unique to you. It may be that raw foods, fruit juices or overly sweetened or processed foods are your triggers. Removing the culprits is then a matter of planning. You may find that after some time away from triggers, you can re-introduce them in smaller quantities or on isolated occasions, and not experience symptoms. If stress triggers your digestive disturbances, this is slightly harder to manage (see August chapter).

Lacking in acid?

The digestion of food begins in the mouth, with chewing and the enzymes contained in saliva. Much of the digestion of protein takes place in the stomach, where food can remain for several hours. The acid environment in this part of the digestive tract is important both for digestion, and for defence against bacteria.

Acid indigestion is a common problem, but it may be that it is not in fact due to excess acid, but to weakened defences against the acid. Usually, the cells of the stomach are lined with mucus, to protect them from the digestive juices. There is a complex balance between the digestive and protective elements – under the influence of stress, acid production is decreased, and correspondingly, so is the production of mucus. When, for whatever reason, acid production is again increased, the mucus barrier remains thinned, meaning irritation of the stomach lining. Using antacids to soothe the pain signals for the production of even less mucus, and the cycle is perpetuated. Low levels of acid also mean less of a defence against pathogens, and an increased likelihood of infection.

If you suffer from acid reflux, speak to your doctor – you may require investigations. If acid reflux is not a problem, and you have no history of stomach or duodenal ulcer, optimising your stomach acid environment may be helpful, particularly if you feel your digestion to be "slow", or if you feel heavy after protein meals. See a practitioner to discuss the best way to do this. Even those using acid reflux medication may benefit from adding in natural enzymes such as bromelain or papain, to help improve digestion of protein. Improving the stomach acid environment may help ameliorate the symptoms of IBS, reduce the risk of infections and increase the amount of nutrients extracted from food – without sufficient acid, digestion of proteins is not possible.

A bacterium affecting the stomach which can have far-reaching consequences is *H.pylori*. It is involved in the development of gastric and duodenal ulcers, and once detected, can be effectively eradicated with antibiotics - but maintaining a healthy digestive tract, with the beneficial flora and natural acid levels intact decreases the risk of *H. pylori* infection in the first place.

Digestive repair

Reducing intake of the foods which irritate the digestive system will contribute significantly towards allowing the gut to heal itself, and towards helping to reduce troublesome symptoms. Supplements such as glutamine, an amino acid, may be helpful in healing the gut.

Probiotics

Some of the benefits of probiotic supplements have been mentioned in previous chapters. The balance of bacteria in the gut can be affected by stress, diet and infections, and this can impact many aspects of health, aside from digestive health. Quite how gut flora can influence seemingly disparate aspects of health is not yet fully understood, but the fatty acids produced by the bacteria may have a role to play. They have an effect on the chemicals required to regulate the immune system, which has a number of downstream effects, e.g., autoimmune diseases.

Probiotic supplements are in essence live bacteria, so choose a product that states its dose and expiry date. They can be combined with prebiotics, which are the foodstuffs preferred by the "good" bacteria, and supplementing with prebiotics alone, to encourage the "good bacteria" is another option. Avoid commercial "probiotic" drinks – the dose of active bacteria is often low, and these products are rich in sugar.

A clear advantage of maintaining a healthy population of good bacteria is that there is less scope for pathogenic bacteria to invade the gut. Probiotics can be particularly useful supplements when travelling abroad, and after antibiotic therapy.

Fibre

Refined foods were once a luxury, only affordable for a small part of the population – now they make up the base for much of the Western diet. The human gut did not evolve to deal with easy to digest foodstuffs, and so it is no surprise that constipation is a common complaint.

Simply including more natural foods and drinking more water can help to improve the passage of digested foods through the bowel. But where years of poor eating habits have miseducated the digestive system, other measures may be necessary. Prunes and their juice, psyllium husk and senna are all natural approaches to relieving constipation. Including more vegetable fibre in the diet can also be useful (in the form of supplements if necessary), but overuse of bran may be counterproductive as it may further miseducate the gut.

Alcohol

The culture in the UK centres heavily on alcohol. In some professions, heavy drinking is almost expected, and not joining the team and overindulging can lead to feelings of marginalisation.

It is not necessary to cut out alcohol entirely during the festive season, but reducing intake can make sticking to fat loss and wellbeing initiatives much easier. Alcohol produces disinhibition, which leads to poor food choices and potentially overconsumption. Hangovers the following day often mean reduced activity levels, and further poor food choices.

Alcohol addiction and extremely heavy drinking can be fatal. But even on a much lower level, regular alcohol intake above or around the recommended level can be problematic for health – it halts fat loss, stresses the liver and increases the risk of accidents as well as of breast cancer and oro-pharyngeal cancers. Small, regular intakes of wine can be helpful for health – wine contains the powerful phytochemical resveratrol, which has a variety of benefits; wine can be useful in reducing cardiovascular risk.

Consider the following:

- Do you enjoy drinking alcohol?
- Do you enjoy being drunk?
- Do you often regret drinking so much the next day?
- Do you drink in order to not be left out, or because it is expected?

If you like alcoholic drinks, or the occasional opportunity to "let your hair down", then drink in moderation this season. If you do not like the taste of alcoholic drinks, tending to choose sweet alcoholic drinks to mask the taste, dislike being drunk, regretting the experience the next day, or only drink out of habit or because it is expected at particular occasions, you may benefit from changing your patterns. Standing up to pressure from others is not always easy, so you may wish to volunteer to be the driver on evenings out, think of "excuses" or nurse one drink for the whole evening.

Consider the Mediterranean model of consumption – eat, drink and take your time, interspersing alcoholic drinks with water. For each unit of alcohol (half glass of wine, half pint of beer, shot of spirit), have at least 1 glass of water. Avoid mixing types of alcoholic drinks, and steer clear of sweet cocktails and alcopops.

Have a restorative festive season

An ideal Christmas involves enjoyable company, delicious food, happy children. The reality is usually different, with family squabbles, tantrums and feelings of exhaustion.

If you are in charge of organising the festivities for your family or group of friends, book in opportunities to relax. This might mean a massage or beauty treatment, or relaxing alone outdoors. With a little planning and consideration, this can be a truly restorative period. Enjoy!

Chapter summary

- The festive season provides ample opportunities for overindulgence - being aware of how you view food can allow you to have a healthier holiday, without feeling deprived
- Keep a food and symptoms diary, and be kind to your gut - identifying foods that irritate your digestion can mean fewer IBS-type symptoms
- Relax with alcohol if you enjoy it, but beware of drinking just to fit in with tradition, and of giving in to pressure at parties

Workbook section

List some typical festive season activities, how these make you feel, whether you should include them this year and some ideas for alternative activities/solutions.

For example:

Activity: Buying expensive presents for family

How this makes me feel: Worried about finances, obliged

Should I include it this year: Ideally not

Ideas for alternatives: Agree with some family members not to buy presents, make home made gifts, look out for special offers at spas to give as gifts

Review of the year

Changes I have made this year:

What I feel these have achieved for me:

What I would like to do next year:

Resources

The following lists cover online stockists, sources of information and registers of practitioners. They are intended as a starting point, and are not exhaustive, or the only sources of information. I have attempted to include a range of sites, and inclusion on the list does not necessary mean I endorse the associated products or approaches.

Illustrations and artwork
Chris Lyon (created the illustrations for this book)
lyonchristine@hotmail.com

Supplements
Charles Poliquin's website:
www.charlespoliquin.com

Nutri:
www.nutri.co.uk

The Nutri Centre:
www.nutricentre.com

Myprotein - low cost supplements:
myprotein.co.uk

Where to find practitioners
Medical practitioners:
www.gmc-uk.org

NHS Directory of Complementary and Alternative Practitioners:
www.nhsdirectory.org

National Register of Personal Trainers:
www.nrpt.com

The Institute of Sport and Remedial Massage:
www.theisrm.com

The Association of Traditional Chinese Medicine (UK):
www.atcm.co.uk

The Register of Chinese Herbal Medicine
www.rhcm.co.uk

British Acupuncture Council:
www.acupuncture.org.uk

General Osteopathy Council:
www.osteopathy.org.uk

The General Council and Register of Naturopaths
www.naturopathy.org.uk

National Institute of Medical Herbalists
www.nimh.org.uk

Pampering and spa deals
www.wahanda.com
www.livingsocial.com
www.groupon.co.uk

January
NHS guide to weight loss with ideas for workouts: http://www.nhs.uk/Livewell/loseweight/Pages/Tenminuteworkouts.aspx

WebMD tips on home workouts:
http://www.webmd.boots.com/fitness-exercise/guide/6-ways-build-better-body-budget

When choosing a gym, consider the following:

- Value for money – sports centres can offer great facilities at a fraction of the price of chains. Also check out low cost options such as www.thegymgroup.com, but bear in mind that paying a little extra can work out as better value in the long term, depending on your goals and needs
- Convenience – to train at least 3 times per week, the gym needs to be easily accessible from home or work. With some gym companies, a membership entitles you to use any branch within a given area, which may be useful if you travel frequently, or work in different locations
- Type of gym – some gyms include cafes and spas – if you are unlikely to use these facilities, consider something more basic
- Equipment available – a good gym should have a variety of free weights and resistance machines, as well as cardio-vascular workout machines. Many gym chains boast dozens of cardiovascular machines, but a very small free weights area that can quickly become crowded
- Personnel – If you are interested in Personal Training, find out what qualifications the trainers have. Check what is available to you when you join a gym – in some gyms you are entitled to several sessions with a Personal Trainer as part of your membership/joining fee
- You might prefer to train exclusively with a particular Personal Trainer at a Personal Training studio. These are purpose-designed locations for Personal Training only, it is not usually possible to use the facilities without a trainer being present. A well equipped studio should allow free

weights work outs, and not focus only on high intensity cardiovascular work. Enquire about how many clients will be training at any one time, to make sure that you won't end up exercising in a crowded space, and check that times available for training will be convenient for you on an ongoing basis

February

Information on adrenal fatigue:
www.adrenalfatigue.org

Alternative approach to thyroid problems:
The Great Thyroid Scandal and How to Survive It,
Barry Durrant-Peatfield
Barons Down Publishing, 2002
978-0954420307

March

The Dukan Diet:
www.dukandiet.co.uk

The Atkins Diet:
www.atkins.com

Intermittent Fasting:
www.leangains.com

April

Better You magnesium oil for sleep:
www.betteryou.uk.com

May

Information on family planning:
www.foresight-preconception.org.uk

Persona Hormone Monitor:
http://www.persona.org.uk/uk/index.php

Skincare:
www.dermalogica.com/uk
www.skinceuticals.co.uk
www.paiskincare.com

Discount stockist:
www.johnandginger.co.uk

Nourkrin:
www.nourkrin4women.com

June

The Paleo diet:
www.thepaleodiet.com

Basic information on sports injuries:
www.sportsinjuryclinic.net

July

Discussions of UK sun policy and vitamin D. There are books available for download on the site:
www.healthresearchforum.org.uk

Environmental working group - sunscreen:
www.ewg.org/2010sunscreen

Cancer Research UK:
www.sunsmart.org.uk

The Mole Clinic - information on skin cancer and services for mole checking www.themoleclinic.co.uk

August

The Cortisol Connection
Shawn Talbott
Hunter House, 2007
978-0897934923

UK NLP resource
www.anlp.org

Farm direct delivery service
www.farm-direct.com

Able and Cole delivery service
www.abelandcole.co.uk

Riverford delivery service
www.riverford.co.uk

Farmers markets
www.farmersmarkets.net

Seasonal eating
Paul Waddington, Eden House Project Books, 2004
978-1903919521

October

SAD resources
www.sad.org.uk – includes details of recommended manufacturers
www.sada.org.uk
www.lumie.com
www.sadbox.co.uk

www.realsunlight.co.uk – equipment for providing nature-identical light, with harmful UV removed
www.negativeions.com

Bibliography/ Further Reading

Books

Animal, Vegetable, Miracle
Barbara Kingsolver
Faber and Faber, 2008
978-0571233571

Eat, Drink and Be Gorgeous
Esther Blum
Chronicle Books, 2007
978-0811855402

Good Calories, Bad Calories
Gary Taubes
Anchor Books, 2008
978-1-4000-3346-1

Healing with the Herbs of Life
Lesley Tierra
Crossing Press, 2003
978-1-58091-147-4

In Defence of Food
Michael Pollan
Penguin, 2009
978-0141034720

Molecules of Emotion
Candace B Pert
Pocket Books, 1999
978-0671033972

Outliers: The Story of Success
Michael Gladwell
Penguin, 2009
978-0141036250

Textbook of Functional Medicine
Institute for Functional Medicine (David S Jones, Editor in Chief), 2006
978-0-90773713-0-3

The Stations of the Sun - A History of the Ritual Year in Britain
Ronald Hutton
Oxford University Press, 1996
0-19-820570-8

Why Do People Get Ill?
Darian Leader and David Corfield
Penguin 2008
978-0141021218

Papers

Dairy

A prospective study of dairy foods intake and anovulatory infertility
Chavarro JE *et al.*,Hum Reprod. 2007 May;22(5):1340-7. Epub 2007 Feb 28
Dairy products, calcium and the risk of breast cancer: results of the French SU.VI.MAX prospective study
Kesse-Guyot E *et al.*, Ann Nutr Metab. 2007;51(2):139-45

Dairy product consumption and the risk of breast cancer
Parodi PW *et al.*, J Am Coll Nutr. 2005 Dec;24(6 Suppl):556S-68S

Dairy products and breast cancer: the IGF-I, estrogen, and bGH hypothesis
Outwater JL *et al.*,Med Hypotheses. 1997 Jun;48(6):453-61

The experience of Japan as a clue to the etiology of breast and ovarian cancers: relationship between death from both malignancies and dietary practices
Li XM *et al.*, Med Hypotheses. 2003 Feb;60(2):268-75

Nutrition and acne
Danby FW, Clin Dermatol. 2010 Nov-Dec;28(6):598-604

Acne, dairy and cancer: The 5alpha-P link
Danby FW, Dermatoendocrinol. 2009 Jan;1(1):12-6

Depression

Blood serotonin, serum melatonin and light therapy in healthy subjects and in patients with nonseasonal depression
Rao ML *et al.*, Acta Psychiatr Scand. 1992 Aug;86(2):127-32

A randomized, placebo-controlled trial of bright light and high-density negative air ions for treatment of Seasonal Affective Disorder
Flory R *et al.*, Psychiatry Res. 2010 May 15;177(1-2):101-8

Second-tier natural antidepressants: Review and critique
Iovieno N *et al.*, J Affect Disord. 2010 Jun 24

The evidence base of complementary and alternative therapies in depression
Thachil AF et al., J Affect Disord. 2007 Jan;97(1-3):23-35

Herbal remedies

Possible mechanisms of dose-dependent cough suppressive effect of

Althaea officinalis rhamnogalacturonan in guinea pigs test system
Sutovská M *et al.*, Int J Biol Macromol. 2009 Jul 1;45(1):27-32

Effect of enzymatically modified isoquercitrin, a flavonoid, on symptoms of Japanese cedar pollinosis: a randomized double-blind placebo-controlled trial
Kawai M *et al.*, Int Arch Allergy Immunol. 2009;149(4):359-68

Evaluation of echinacea for the prevention and treatment of the common cold: a meta-analysis
Shah SA *et al.* Lancet Infect Dis. 2007 Jul;7(7):473-80

Valerian-hops combination and diphenhydramine for treating insomnia: a randomized placebo-controlled clinical trial
Morin *et al.*, Sleep. 2005 Nov 1;28(11):1465-71

Extract of Perilla frutescens enriched for rosmarinic acid, a polyphenolic phytochemical, inhibits seasonal allergic rhinoconjunctivitis in humans
Takano H *et al.*, Exp Biol Med (Maywood). 2004 Mar;229(3):247-54

Potent inhibition of human phosphodiesterase-5 by icariin derivatives
Dell'Agli M *et al.*, J Nat Prod. 2008 Sep;71(9):1513-7

Short- and long-term effects of Ginkgo biloba extract on sexual dysfunction in women
Meston CM *et al.*, Arch Sex Behav. 2008 Aug;37(4):530-47

The effect of five weeks of Tribulus terrestris supplementation on muscle strength and body composition during preseason training in elite rugby league players
Rogerson S *et al.*, J Strength Cond Res. 2007 May;21(2):348-53

A pilot investigation into the effect of maca supplementation on physical activity and sexual desire in sportsmen
Stone M *et al.*, J Ethnopharmacol. 2009 Dec 10;126(3):574-6

Treatment for the premenstrual syndrome with agnus castus fruit extract: prospective, randomised, placebo controlled study
Schellenberg R, BMJ. 2001 Jan 20;322(7279):134-7

A randomised, double-blind, placebo-controlled, parallel-group study of the standardised extract shr-5 of the roots of Rhodiola rosea in the treatment of subjects with stress-related fatigue
Olsson EM *et al.*, Planta Med. 2009 Feb;75(2):105-12

Withania somnifera improves semen quality by regulating reproductive hormone levels and oxidative stress in seminal plasma of infertile males
Ahmad MK *et al.*, Fertil Steril. 2010 Aug;94(3):989-96

Antimicrobial activity of oleanolic acid from Salvia officinalis and related compounds on vancomycin-resistant enterococci (VRE)
Horiuchi K *et al.*, Biol Pharm Bull. 2007 Jun;30(6):1147-9

Omega-3

Omega-3 polyunsaturated fatty acids and immune-mediated diseases: inflammatory bowel disease and rheumatoid arthritis
Ruggiero *et al.*, Curr Pharm Des. 2009;15(36):4135-48

Omega-3 fatty acids: cardiovascular benefits, sources and sustainability
Lee JH *et al.*, Nat Rev Cardiol. 2009 Dec;6(12):753-8

The role of omega-3 fatty acids in mood disorders
Stahl *et al.*, Curr Opin Investig Drugs. 2008 Jan;9(1):57-64

Probiotics/Synbiotics

Specific probiotics alleviate allergic rhinitis during the birch pollen season
Ouwehand AC *et al.*, World J Gastroenterol. 2009 Jul 14;15(26):3261-8

Effect of konjac glucomannan hydrolysates and probiotics on the growth of the skin bacterium Propionibacterium acnes in vitro
Al-Ghazzewi FH, Tester RF, Int J Cosmet Sci. 2010 Apr;32(2):139-42

Probiotics in gastrointestinal disorders
Quigley EM, Hosp Pract (Minneap). 2010 Nov;38(4):122-9

Probiotic effects on cold and influenza-like symptom incidence and duration in children
Leyer GJ *et al.*, Pediatrics. 2009 Aug;124(2):e172-9

A new chance of preventing winter diseases by the administration of synbiotic formulations
Pregliasco F *et al.*, J Clin Gastroenterol. 2008 Sep;42 Suppl 3 Pt 2:S224-33

Vitamins

Short-term folate, vitamin B-12 or vitamin B-6 supplementation slightly affects memory performance but not mood in women of various ages
Bryan J *et al.*, J Nutr. 2002 Jun;132(6):1345-56

Effects of high-dose B vitamin complex with vitamin C and minerals on subjective mood and performance in healthy males
Kennedy DO *et al.*, Psychopharmacology (Berl). 2010 Jul;211(1):55-68

Treatment of depression: time to consider folic acid and vitamin B12
Coppen A, Bolander-Gouaille C, J Psychopharmacol. 2005 Jan;19(1):59-65

Vitamin C for preventing and treating the common cold
Douglas *et al.*, Cochrane Database Syst Rev. 2007 Jul 18;(3):CD000980

Vitamin D and breast cancer risk
Colston KW, Best Pract Res Clin Endocrinol Metab. 2008 Aug;22(4):587-99

Vitamin D and breast cancer
Bertone-Johnson ER, Ann Epidemiol. 2009 Jul;19(7):462-7

Vitamin D and prostate cancer risk: a review of the epidemiological literature
Gupta D *et al.*, Prostate Cancer Prostatic Dis. 2009;12(3):215-26

Vitamin D and cardiovascular disease risk
Michos ED, Melamed ML, Curr Opin Clin Nutr Metab Care. 2008 Jan;11(1):7-12

Vitamin D in Atopic Dermatitis, Asthma and Allergic Diseases
Searing DA, Leung DY, Immunol Allergy Clin North Am. 2010 Aug;30(3):397-409

Maternal vitamin D intake during pregnancy is inversely associated with asthma and allergic rhinitis in 5-year-old children
Erkkola *et al.*, Clin Exp Allergy. 2009 Jun;39(6):875-82

Relation of schizophrenia prevalence to latitude, climate, fish consumption, infant mortality, and skin color: a role for prenatal vitamin d deficiency and infections?

Kinney DK *et al.*, Schizophr Bull. 2009 May;35(3):582-95

Vitamin D status, 1,25-dihydroxyvitamin D3, and the immune system
Cantorna et al, Am J Clin Nutr. 2004 Dec;80(6 Suppl):1717S-20S

Assessment of evidence for a protective role of vitamin D in multiple sclerosis
Hanwell HE, Banwell B, Biochim Biophys Acta. 2010 Jul 29

Other

The influence of painful sunburns and lifetime sun exposure on the risk of actinic keratoses, seborrheic warts, melanocytic nevi, atypical nevi, and skin cancer
Kennedy C *et al.*, J Invest Dermatol. 2003 Jun;120(6):1087-93

Feed a cold, starve a fever?
van den Brink GR *et al.*, Clin Diagn Lab Immunol. 2002 Jan;9(1):182-3

Immune system of cold-exposed and cold-adapted humans
Janský L *et al.*, Eur J Appl Physiol Occup Physiol. 1996;72(5-6):445-50

Researchers find no sperm in pre-ejaculate fluid
Contracept Technol Update. 1993 Oct;14(10):154-6

Double-blind, randomised, placebo-controlled study to evaluate the efficacy and safety of a fixed combination containing two plant extracts (Crataegus oxyacantha and Eschscholtzia californica) and magnesium in mild-to-moderate anxiety disorders
Hanus M *et al.*, Curr Med Res Opin. 2004 Jan;20(1):63-71

Association between magnesium intake and depression and anxiety in community-dwelling adults: the Hordaland Health Study

Jacka FN *et al.*, Aust N Z J Psychiatry. 2009 Jan;43(1):45-52

Chronopathological forms of magnesium depletion with hypofunction or with hyperfunction of the biological clock
Durlach J *et al.*, Magnes Res. 2002 Dec;15(3-4):263-8

Vitamin E and evening primrose oil for management of cyclical mastalgia: a randomized pilot study
Pruthi S *et al.*, Altern Med Rev. 2010 Apr;15(1):59-67

Social relationships and mortality risk: a meta-analytic review
Holt-Lunstad J *et al.*, PLoS Med. 2010 Jul 27;7(7):e1000316

Normalization of leaky gut in chronic fatigue syndrome (CFS) is accompanied by a clinical improvement: effects of age, duration of illness and the translocation of LPS from gram-negative bacteria
Maes M, Leunis JC, Neuro Endocrinol Lett. 2008 Dec;29(6):902-10

Benefits and risks of sauna bathing
Hannuksela ML, Ellahham S, Am J Med. 2001 Feb 1;110(2):118-26

Endonasal phototherapy significantly alleviates symptoms of allergic rhinitis, but has a limited impact on the nasal mucosal immune cells.
Brehmer D, Schön MP, Eur Arch Otorhinolaryngol. 2010 Sep 3

Pilot study of the efficacy and safety of a modified-release magnesium 250 mg tablet (Sincromag) for the treatment of premenstrual syndrome
Quaranta S *et al.*, Clin Drug Investig. 2007;27(1):51-8

A randomized, placebo-controlled trial of an amino acid preparation on timing and quality of sleep

Shell W et al., Am J Ther. 2010 Mar-Apr;17(2):133-9

5-Hydroxytryptophan: a clinically-effective serotonin precursor
Birdsall TC, Altern Med Rev. 1998 Aug;3(4):271-80

Effects of oral L: -carnitine supplementation on insulin sensitivity indices in response to glucose feeding in lean and overweight/obese males
Galloway SD *et al.*, Amino Acids. 2010 Oct 21
Carnitine insufficiency caused by aging and overnutrition compromises mitochondrial performance and metabolic control
Noland RC, J Biol Chem. 2009 Aug 21;284(34):22840-52

The effects of oral glutamine supplementation on athletes after prolonged, exhaustive exercise
Castell LM, Newsholme EA, Nutrition. 1997 Jul-Aug;13(7-8):738-42

Glutamine supplementation decreases intestinal permeability and preserves gut mucosa integrity in an experimental mouse model
dos Santos RG et al., JPEN J Parenter Enteral Nutr. 2010 Jul-Aug;34(4):408-13

Whole- and refined-grain intakes are differentially associated with abdominal visceral and subcutaneous adiposity in healthy adults: the Framingham Heart Study
McKeown NM et al., Am J Clin Nutr. 2010 Nov;92(5):1165-71